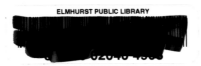
"Infertility is painful. In these pages, Matthew Arbo gives biblical insight and wise counsel, offering both comfort and hope for those on this difficult journey. *Walking through Infertility* goes deeper than the superficial clichés couples often hear, which, though intended to comfort, can hurt. Arbo frames infertility within the biblical narrative, where it is actually quite common and significant—we find we are not alone. Additionally, he helps those navigating some of the complex ethical decisions made possible by modern technology for dealing with infertility—we are not without guidance. Ultimately, he points to our comfort in the community of the church and our hope in the God of life."

Joshua Ryan Butler, Pastor, Imago Dei Community,
Portland, Oregon; author, *The Skeletons in God's Closet* and
The Pursuing God

"I am glad to commend Matthew Arbo's *Walking through Infertility* both to couples going down this road and to the friends, family members, and professionals who walk this road with them. It is sensitively done, and full of wisdom and insight about what these couples are facing. It's a worthwhile resource, which I will often consult."

Scott B. Rae, Professor of Christian Ethics, Talbot School of
Theology, Biola University

"*Walking through Infertility* is a resource I wish had been available when we walked through our own struggles with infertility. In an age of increasing medical advancement, the options for couples are numerous and often overwhelming. Matthew Arbo has provided a helpful resource for couples as they consider what the Bible has to say about infertility and how God's Word speaks to the various treatments out there. But Arbo also speaks to church leaders, who are often left wondering how to counsel those under their care. This is a needed book, and I'm glad it's finally here."

Courtney Reissig, author, *Glory in the Ordinary* and
The Accidental Feminist

D1506215

"The challenges of infertility raise serious and substantive pastoral and ethical questions, yet few accessible—much less biblical—volumes exist to address them. Matthew Arbo's sensitive and careful discussion is alive to the struggles couples face, yet concerned about the ethical temptations that arise within them. This is a helpful volume, with theologically grounded counsel that lay leaders and pastors should weigh carefully."

Matthew Lee Anderson, Founder, Mere Orthodoxy; author, *The End of Our Exploring: A Book about Questioning and the Confidence of Faith*

WALKING
through
INFERTILITY

WALKING
through
INFERTILITY

BIBLICAL, THEOLOGICAL,
AND MORAL COUNSEL FOR
THOSE WHO ARE STRUGGLING

MATTHEW ARBO

Foreword by Karen Swallow Prior

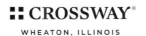

:: CROSSWAY®

WHEATON, ILLINOIS

Trade paperback ISBN: 978-1-4335-5931-0
ePub ISBN: 978-1-4335-5934-1
PDF ISBN: 978-1-4335-5932-7
Mobipocket ISBN: 978-1-4335-5933-4

Library of Congress Cataloging-in-Publication Data

Names: Arbo, Matthew, 1981– author.
Title: Walking through infertility : biblical, theological, and moral counsel for those who are struggling / Matthew Arbo.
Description: Wheaton : Crossway, 2018. | Includes bibliographical references and index.
Identifiers: LCCN 2017057938 (print) | LCCN 2018020306 (ebook) | ISBN 9781433559327 (pdf) | ISBN 9781433559334 (mobi) | ISBN 9781433559341 (epub) | ISBN 9781433559310 (tp)
Subjects: LCSH: Infertility—Patients—Counseling of—Moral and ethical aspects. | Infertility—Religious aspects. | Infertility—Psychological aspects.
Classification: LCC RC889 (ebook) | LCC RC889 .A67 2018 (print) | DDC 616.6/920651—dc23
LC record available at https://lccn.loc.gov/2017057938

Crossway is a publishing ministry of Good News Publishers.

BP		28	27	26	25	24	23	22	21	20	19	18
15	14	13	12	11	10	9	8	7	6	5	4	3	2	1

To Patrick and Jennifer

Contents

Foreword

Karen Swallow Prior

I'll never forget the moment I realized that I hadn't been given the gift of musicality.

As the granddaughter of an accomplished bandmaster and the daughter of a lifelong choir singer, I was six when, immediately upon showing an interest, I was started on piano lessons. For years, I had weekly instruction and practiced daily at home on our old wooden upright.

One afternoon, I arrived at my piano teacher's house early and sat in the foyer to await the end of the session of the student ahead of me. The girl was a year older than me, but I knew she'd been taking lessons for less time than I had. Sitting quietly by myself, listening to her play, I noticed a smoothness and gracefulness in her notes I had never heard from my own fingers. In that instant, I recognized for the first time that—not for any lack of trying or desire—I truly lacked musical talent. Suddenly, I felt free. I was but a teenager, but I had figured out on my own what no one else seemed able to see or willing to say.

I quit piano lessons and took up cross country. I've been running ever since.

My journey through infertility replicated this experience in significant ways.

Like most women, I desired from a young age to become a mother someday and assumed that I would. Everyone around me, particularly in our church life, appeared to share this assumption. When my husband and I didn't conceive right away, everyone seemingly assumed we would follow the prescribed course for most infertile couples, partaking of increasingly invasive and risky procedures until pregnancy was achieved. No one advised us to stop and consider that perhaps God simply wasn't going to give us the gift of children. But my husband had the wisdom to apply the brakes. Yes, we desired the gift of children—but we weren't willing to create life in ways that we believe risk harm to that life. Notably, the verse in Psalms that proclaims that children are a gift of the Lord (127:3) is preceded two verses before with the caution, "Unless the Lord builds the house, those who build it labor in vain" (Ps. 127:1).

Not long after we were married, a family member gave me some of her old maternity clothes, baby clothes, and a fold-up stroller. Unquestioningly, I took them home and packed them safely away for someday. Because it was a long time before my husband and I learned that we were infertile, we dutifully lugged these items around for years, from apartment to apartment, where they took up scant closet space, before eventually giving them away to someone who could actually use them. It was even longer before I realized what a burden that baggage had been. And I don't mean the baby supplies. The real baggage was the presumption that every godly family follows the same course and achieves the same standard outcome.

God's design for the family—the fruitful marriage between a man and a woman, the union of two image bearers that brings forth more image bearers—is mysterious, wonderful, and good. To desire such is good. Both marriage and children are God's good gifts. But to assume that God will give certain gifts is not good. Nor is it good to cultivate within the church the presumption that God is going to give his gifts to everyone—just as surely as I won't be accompanying next week's soloist at the piano.

To have one's longing to marry and have children go unmet is, as with any frustrated desire, disappointing. However, the depth of that disappointment can be increased even beyond what is natural with the additional imposition of expectations—whether others' or our own.

As Matt writes in the following pages, "Every experience of infertility is a storied experience. . . .Through story we situate ourselves and others to help make sense of where we are and how we got here." The fact is that what we think is the standard story for the family is more culturally influenced than we realize. Indeed, in many chapters of church history, beginning with the apostle Paul, marriage and family have not been the assumed norm for those devoted to lives of service to Christ. The power of the stories we tell ourselves—based on the story given to us by our culture—can be positive, but it can also be destructive. The prevailing narrative within the culture, church culture included, that assumes family life looks a particular way and follows a certain path conditions those who don't adhere to that plot to feel, wrongly, out of place in the story. Recognizing those pressures for what they are will not, of course, eliminate entirely the sense of suffering and loss that comes when our personal desires are thwarted. However, embracing the understanding that life doesn't always (nor does it have to) look one way in order to please God and be fulfilling can go a long way in guiding our responses to frustrated expectations and desires.

Matt wisely writes that "*the Creator and Redeemer of life has not forsaken the infertile but has instead given them a slightly different way of being family and thus of participating in the life and mission of God.*" Imagine what the church would look like if infertile couples were taught, discipled, and encouraged in the knowledge that God has other plans for their earthly ministry, and if the church equipped them to find and carry out those plans. Some of these couples might be called to adopt children. Some might be called to devote time to other members of their families. Some might be called to serve the kingdom through church ministry, intentional communities, creative artistry, or secular vocations.

Another part of this picture we might envision is what a church that purposefully makes space for childless women to offer the gifts of their minds, mothering, and time would look like. Not only might infertile women feel a bit less the burden of longing, loss, and shame that often accompany infertility, but the church would be richer in cultivating and receiving the gifts such women have been given. I'm thankful this has been my own experience in the church. But I lament that this experience for infertile women is not universal.

May this book help make it so.

Introduction

A Modern Story of Infertility

John and Lizzy first met at a student ministry gathering at their college in Colorado. It was serendipitous in the way so many comedic first-meets are. They were crazy for one another from the start. Infatuated. Inseparable. They had everything in common. A short year later, to no one's surprise, they were engaged. He studied engineering; she studied journalism. They married in a small chapel in the Rocky Mountain foothills not many weeks after graduation. Parents wept, friends cheered, and the felicitous couple laughed their way through the first few years of marriage. And although they never really put it to themselves this way, both John and Lizzy felt deep down that everything in life had really gone according to plan. They were on their way together and figured at some point a gaggle of children would soon follow.

Seven years later, childless, John and Lizzy's once raucous joy had stilled, and their hopeful expectations were all but muted by loneliness. When they ceased using contraceptives shortly after their third anniversary, they naturally assumed conception was imminent. But failing to conceive after six or seven cycles, Lizzy became anxious: was there some biological problem?

She discussed her nervousness with John over the next month or so and decided to schedule an appointment with her obstetrician. She was pleased she did. The OB instructed her to pay even closer attention to her natural cycle and to have intercourse with her husband every day she was at her most fertile. Her doctor also recommended some additional blood and hormonal testing, which to Lizzy's surprise revealed a slight imbalance in estrogen, comparably easy to treat. Things were looking up again. This little imbalance must have been the problem all along. Nevertheless, despite implementing a rigorous sexual itinerary and treatment regimen, ten months later John and Lizzy still hadn't conceived. And everywhere they were reminded of the fact.

The new impasse meant it was John's turn for assessment. He and Lizzy were referred to a well-known fertility specialist and, following a battery of tests, John was given a clean bill of reproductive health. Nothing on John's end seemed to be preventing conception. Results that should have been relieving were, in their case, crushing in their implications. They could not conceive, and the hidden reason had something to do with their bodies. It all felt deeply indicting.

Anxiety was assuaged somewhat by the specialist's immediate rejoinder: there was still hope. It was time to try a new, more involved phase of treatment. Lizzy would undergo a fresh series of scans and screenings. They would get to the bottom of this, he told them. It would be expensive and laborious, but it was the only way forward if they wished to have a biological child.

In Vitro Fertilization: IVF. They had read a bit about the procedure in online forums for couples experiencing infertility. It seemed feasible for them on first glance, and they were certainly ideal candidates. But the sticker shock! They were still paying off college loans. And they had purchased their first home only the year before. The savings just weren't there yet.

Quite apart from the financial concern, they also harbored reservations about the ethics of the procedure itself. Its clinical artificiality and transactional character rubbed their consciences wrong, although they couldn't quite say why. IVF appealed to them, in a way, but they would need some time to evaluate their options. Maybe adoption made more sense for them. Or perhaps embryo adoption, which they'd begun to hear more and more about from random friends online, was something they should consider. Whatever they ultimately decided, they'd need more money, wisdom, and time to make it happen.

Through it all, from the earliest days of subtle worry to the later seasons of empty bedrooms and indelicate conversations at church, John and Lizzy felt the full range of emotions that attend the experience of infertility. Eagerness, worry, hope, disappointment, confidence, despair, embarrassment—they felt it all—and always, everywhere the irrepressible *shame* of not being able to complete the basic human task of reproduction. It was an irrational feeling, they knew, and yet they couldn't fully banish it from their hearts. It had fastened itself to them. Shame dug at them with every opportunity—children bounding loudly on playgrounds, toddlers chuckling in shopping carts, birth announcements arriving in the mail, baby dedications at church—they couldn't escape the reproach.

Inevitably the shame hardened into bitter anger each took out on the other. That's often the nature of infertility, the "fault" is either his or hers. Human beings are pathological about wanting to fix responsibility for a problem. The trouble with this tendency is that fixing responsibility tends in reality to result in *blaming*. John and Lizzy took their turns with each other. Blaming became an almost daily venting ritual. At its worst, they both at different times wondered to themselves whether it would be better to leave and chart a new life with someone else, far away from the hell their life together had descended into. At its best, well, as far as they could tell, there really was no "best."

Where We're Going

John and Lizzy's story will pick up again in the next chapter. Even though their story is not characteristic of every infertile couple's experience, or even yours, it nevertheless is the story of tens of thousands of infertile couples. It is the story of your friends and family. Our stories have their own variations, of course—different characters, plot points, settings, responses, and conclusions. Not everyone responds to infertility in the same way as John and Lizzy. Each couple facing infertility responds to specific turns of events in their own way. It's better to think of infertility as having no one type, but as sitting somewhere on a spectrum, or range of possible events and reactions.

The Centers for Disease Control estimates approximately 7 to 10 percent of all couples experience some form of reproductive infertility. For some of these couples surgical intervention or other less invasive treatments fix the problem, and they are subsequently able to conceive. For others, however, infertility is an untreatable biological fact. Infertile couples often begin with the expectation that their condition is reparable, that some medical solution will resolve the problems preventing conception or gestation. The confidence of that assumption weakens over time. The longer infertility is protracted, the more likely a couple will resort to extrabodily (i.e., artificial) treatments to ensure the birth of a biological child. For some couples, prolonged reproductive treatment is entirely cost prohibitive.

Infertility is often a profoundly wounding experience for many couples. The temptation is for husband or wife to become intensely self-critical and to view themselves as somehow responsible for their plight. As a result, they feel hurt or perhaps even ashamed by their infertility. They blame God. They do not know exactly what to say to others. Even when they do, the response from friends and family, however well-meaning, is often timid and ignorant. Couples sometimes assume their fertile peers look down upon them. And if childlessness itself were not enough, the social castigation, even if unreal and imagined by the couple, often carries significant emotional trauma.

The purpose of this book is to address biblical, theological, and moral questions surrounding infertility. The aim is to instruct and inspire the church, especially those couples with personal experience with infertility. If you're reading this, chances are you've thought about some of these questions. But I want to do more than instruct you—I want to encourage you. I want you to hear and receive the truth, and I want to extend some words of hope and consolation: *God is present to you.* His grace is sufficient.

We'll begin first by rehearsing some the Bible's infertility narratives. The purpose of these stories is not necessarily to illustrate the hardship of infertility or to promise God's certain answer. It is more complicated than that. These narratives do, however, reveal that God cares about fertility, and we'll want to discern what his caring means for the Christian and for the church.

These biblical cases will serve as a useful backdrop for the second chapter on Christian discipleship and the importance of human affection. How might understanding discipleship illumine our thinking—and feeling—about infertility? That's the question we want to grapple with. Formulating a response will lead us into chapter 3, which explores the vitality and consoling support of the church.

With these biblical and theological themes in place, the final chapter will offer a brief, accessible moral assessment of a few reproductive therapies and treatments sometimes commended to couples experiencing infertility. The moral (and theological) implications of such treatments are not always clear, and medical practitioners do not always unpack those implications transparently for patients. The ethics of reproductive treatment can be inordinately complex. So, moving forward, my aim is to make the moral issues at stake as clear and understandable as possible.

Here's the central idea of this book: *the Creator and Redeemer of life has not forsaken the infertile but has instead given them a slightly different way of being family, and thus of participating in the life and mission of God.* In God is life. He is the only final source of human consolation, for fertile and infertile alike. God is infinitely good. He is wise. We worship an almighty God.

If God does not gift a couple with children of their own progeny, the task for Christian couples is to wait upon the Lord in faith and obedience. This waiting differs dramatically from fatalistic resignation. *Waiting* in Scripture is akin to eager receptivity to God and his Word. It is precisely this waiting that enables the Christian couple to interpret their situation rightly and also to form wise assessments of complex fertility treatments. The moral rightness or wrongness of a treatment, on the Christian theological account, will depend entirely upon whether the treatment corresponds to who God is and to what God has said about the making and taking of life. Sometimes that's just not altogether obvious to us, so we'll need to pray and think and discern a course of action with God's help.

Fear not, I will do everything I can to avoid confusing you or deepening any of your already painful wounds. I'm attempting to be sensitive to the personal experiences of couples who have faced the terrible adversity of infertility. I did not write this book to rebuke you or to remind you all over again of what isn't possible. Nor did I write it simply to give you checklist criteria for evaluating all your medical options. No, this book was written *to help you see and understand that God is the Giver of life.* You are *his* child. He cares deeply about you. When you hurt, he hurts with you.

This book is for infertile couples at all stages, from first worry to full acceptance, and for anyone who wishes to better understand the experience of infertility and to minister to those in the midst of pain. I can't address every discreet variation or every unique eventuality infertile couples may encounter, but I can address some of the general stages and connect them to the purposes of the book. My hope is to offer a picture you can see yourself or others fitting into—a message of hope found in Jesus Christ you can hear and resonate with. So, this book is for infertile couples, for their friends and family, pastors, counselors, or really any Christian who wants to better understand infertility in light of who God is and what he's done. After all, "he is before all things, and in him all things hold together" (Col. 1:17). He is life.

1

Stories of Infertility and God's Abiding Promise

John and Lizzy's frustrations were not restricted to each other, to their marriage, or to their infertility. The few people they let in on their secret often said things that tended to do more harm than good. They were well-meaning, of course. Touched by John or Lizzy's vulnerability, they felt impressed to "speak into their lives," only it scarcely felt to John or Lizzy like words of consolation or counsel, but rather of denial or naiveté. It struck them not as wisdom, but platitudes. "It will happen!" friends would say. "The moment you stop trying so hard, you're sure to get pregnant." Or, "You know, adopting is one of the best fertility treatments, because the pressure of having a child is alleviated and then just like that—a bun in the oven!"

The fact is most people want to help by talking first and talking often. Simply being there for others is much harder. Christians are often no better at "weeping with those who weep" than they are of "rejoicing with those who rejoice" (Rom. 12:15). When John and Lizzy disclosed their experience to others, they were given all varieties of advice—all of it more or less reducible to "cheer up, it'll happen in time." After a few years of this dismissive reassurance, John and Lizzy couldn't help but feel this sort of response was really just an indelicate way of avoiding the real hardship of bearing with someone through the pain of infertility and childlessness.

Throughout their infertility, but especially early on, the ribbing provocation of friends and family discouraged them most. "So, when are you two going to have a baby?" "What are you waiting on?" "Your parents really deserve a grandbaby." "Better while you're young!" Even less empathetic remarks were offered on a semiregular basis. On every occasion they felt an implicit judgment: they do not have children, and should. How were they supposed to respond to such thoughtlessness? They defaulted to their usual politeness, absorbing the rebuke. People just didn't understand what they were saying. Better to keep peace.

John and Lizzy wanted children but could not conceive. That was the problem, not preference or expectation management. They learned gradually the importance of discretion. Not everyone was trustworthy. Not everyone sincerely cared about their experience. They also learned over time how to rest in the peace of Christ. They could do only their part, after all; that which was beyond their power they left to Jesus. They asked him for the virtues and affections needed to persevere. When the words of others were hollow or hurtful, they cleaved to the words of their Savior. He alone was their hope and consolation. In him was *life*.

Where We're Going

Every experience of infertility is a storied experience. Each story has its own characters, setting, and plot. We need stories. Through story we situate ourselves and others to help make sense of where we are and how we got here. It is crucial to our self-understanding that we encounter the stories of others. Hearing others' stories reminds us we are not alone. This is particularly important when it comes to the experience of infertility, as it so naturally fosters a kind of solipsism, where couples feel they are the only ones who struggle with it.

The purpose of this chapter is to explore the reproductive obligations the Bible may, on some readings, impose on couples, and then to explore several of the more prominent infertility narratives in Scripture. It will become clear as we proceed that the gospel speaks to the experience of infertility and childlessness. God's Word is life-giving. His gospel is restorative and liberating, incorporating and commissioning. Jesus is the desire of the nations, the Creator and ruler of all. In him is life.

The Propagation Mandate

"Be fruitful and multiply and fill the earth" (Gen. 1:28). So goes God's command to our first parents, Adam and Eve. The earth needed more human inhabitants. God repeats this imperative to Noah and his family following the flood, telling them to go and repopulate the earth (Gen. 9:7). A human presence on the earth matters to God. He made man with breath and dust, and he directs man to procreate in turn. As issued in Genesis, there isn't an option as to whether the command should be obeyed. The command was normative. It was also expedient. In the ancient world, having children was often a matter of life and death, of producing enough food or defending the tribe from aggressors. Failure to procreate was essentially a neglect of duty.

This particular scriptural command is sometimes referred to as a *propagation mandate*. Having children is something a wedded couple *must* do. The fact that it is an obligation means that a couple either upholds or does not uphold their procreative responsibility. Responsibility just works that way—we do it or we don't. Recognizing this is crucial, because what happens next is sometimes less than obvious to us. We associate upholding or not upholding our obligation as either a success or failure. And when we fail at doing what God commands us to do, we naturally begin to assume that we have displeased God and fallen under his judgment. If it cannot be God's fault, we say to ourselves, then it must be mine (or ours).

Let me offer an important point of clarification here. Couples who are open to having children and who do what they can to conceive but who have not (yet) succeeded in conceiving are *not* violating God's command. Conceiving is not a condition for upholding the command. It is a matter of the heart. The couple intends to have children, wants children, and so also wants to keep the command, but for whatever reason children have not yet come. It isn't that the couple tries to have children *in order* to keep the command either—let us not forget our freedom in Christ under the new covenant—but that in attempting to have children it also happens that they're tracking with the heart of God for humanity.

As people of the new covenant, united this side of Christ's death and resurrection, the duty to procreate has a slightly different purpose and rationale. It has moral and theological force, not legal. Here's what I mean. The Christian couple does not procreate simply to comply with God's requirement, but to bring into the world another recipient of grace, a servant to Christ's body, a worshiper of the Lord Most High. Christian parents bring children into the world so that they, too, might receive and enjoy God's grace. The gift of life is, theologically speaking, also a gift *to the child*. Having children just to comply with an obligation is an example of the legalism Paul warns against throughout his letters.

Procreation is a good and beautiful thing to do, but it is not the only purpose of Christian marriage. Debate over the ends of Christian marriage, how to enumerate and rank them, are perennial for the church, particularly between Catholics and Protestants. According to Catholic social teaching, the principal purpose of marriage is procreation. The natural law written into creation itself establishes a definite, inarguable purpose for marriage; indeed, it is the only holy purpose in sexual intercourse. To elevate any other purpose above it violates God's law. This is why, for example, artificial contraception is impermissible for Catholic couples.

Protestants have tended to understand the purposes of marriage a bit differently. Procreation is a good purpose for sex within Christian marriage, but so too is pleasure, intimacy, and friendship. Sex is instrumentalized only if pleasure is made the highest or exclusive purpose in sex, and that is the Catholic worry. But Protestants have understood sex as being for the higher purpose of intimacy and fidelity, and for which pleasure plays only a part.

The Protestant view was not an invention of the Reformation. As Oliver O'Donovan has argued, Christians of the earliest centuries understood friendship to be the highest purpose in marriage.[1] Marital sex may strengthen the bonds of intimacy, loyalty, and friendship, or it may not. The temptation to misuse or exaggerate the capacity of sex to bridge every gap of intimacy is in our time everywhere on display.

Taking the stress point off of procreation in marital sex and subordinating it to the higher good of friendship has tremendous implications for how we think about infertility. If the purpose of marriage is procreation, then it follows that infertile couples cannot satisfy their highest conjugal purpose. Whether simply *intending* to procreate satisfies their purpose is of little consequence, for if they cannot satisfy their purpose materially by having children, then lesser purposes aspired to will always seem to infertile couples, and to others, as inferior, resulting in moral stratification.

If, on the other hand, procreation is subordinated to the higher good of friendship in Christian marriage, then infertility isn't a failure, but merely a factor of their relationship. Marriage is about more than having children. Indeed, it is about much more than friendship, too. The purpose of Christian marriage, as Paul understood, is mission. Christian marriage bears witness to the good news in Jesus Christ, to the love he extends to his bride, the church. Any children or friendship in marriage are understood in light of *that* purpose, and in turn receive their real meaning.

While on the subject, can't we also identify good and faithful Christian reasons for a couple to delay or refrain (for a time) from having children? It isn't difficult to imagine circumstances arising that might make the sudden arrival of children a physical, financial, or even spiritual hardship. Conception cannot always be perfectly timed or managed, of course, but if it is within a couple's faithful, prudent discretion to postpone having children, then there cannot also be an opposite obligation to have children whenever or however possible.

The exact reasons for delay are crucial. It is one thing, for example, to delay until a couple has saved enough money to pay for a hospital delivery and associated expenses, say, or to work through some sort of personal crisis. But it is quite another thing to delay having children until financial success is achieved, or because children are inconvenient, or some other unconvincing reason. A couple should therefore seek to discern the just, charitable, and prudent conditions for having children. Not, I should stress, the *ideal* conditions. Ideal conditions for having children do not exist! That's a destructive myth. Ignore ideals, and focus instead on God's gracious leading.

It's better to think of having children as a good thing to do, rather than an obligatory thing to do. No one is displeasing God by being unable to conceive. Humans can't be held responsible for not doing what isn't even possible for them to do. All any Christian couple can do is put themselves at God's disposal: to live as disciples, together, receptive to his Word and open to his grace.

With all that said, however, and speaking for a moment to infertile readers, my guess is that infertility isn't hard for you because of some unfulfilled obligation you might feel toward God or society or family or spouse. It is hard because you long so deeply for a child of your own. It is hard because you long to bring a new one into the world you can parent and befriend. It is hard because you imagine a story for yourself—and your family—that includes more characters than you and your spouse. It is hard because becoming a parent seems as though it will redefine your place in the world. It is hard because you want to love a child through to adulthood. It is hard because you want to *be* a mom or dad. It is hard because the absence of a child means you may miss out on profound and enriching experiences reserved only for parent and child. It is hard because you want to hear children laughing, to console their sobs, to share meals with them, to tell them stories. It is hard because you want to fit in, and because you despair at being seen as deficient or less than human. It is hard because you love your spouse and want this for him or her, too. Even if some of these don't quite correspond to your own hopes and disappointments, you can undoubtedly supply your own that do.

It is hard, you realize, both for good and bad reasons. Sometimes you feel rage, and sometimes you feel hopeless. At your lowest, perhaps, you feel alone and confused and forsaken. But may I offer you some reassurance? You are not alone. You are not alone in your experience, nor are you alone when you *feel* alone. A great many other couples have experienced infertility. Infertility is a recurring theme in the book of Genesis, actually. In examining a few of the narratives I want you to keep the following truth in mind: because God is our Father we can be assured that he cares for his children and cares in turn for the childless.

Biblical Narratives

Now that we've given some contours to God's creation and to the command "be fruitful," let's turn our attention to a few biblical narratives that capture the experience of infertility and God's response to that experience. The stories are unique but share some discreet similarities, one of which will prove striking: *God cares for the childless.*

Abram and Sarai (Genesis 15–21). Years have passed since the Lord first covenanted with Abram, promising to bless him and to bless all the families of the earth through him. The boundless hope provoked by Abram's first encounter with the Lord hardens into frustration over time. From Abram's viewpoint, God has been too slow in fulfilling the promise. So, he lodges a complaint with God: "Behold, you have given me no offspring" (15:3). God hears Abram, and promises him innumerable offspring, as many as the stars in the sky. The covenant is reaffirmed.

Time passes, however, and Abram and Sarai still have no children. Sarai proposes an alternate way of securing a family heir. Sleep with her servant, Hagar, she suggests to Abram, and perhaps that will resolve the dilemma. Abram doesn't put up much of a fight to the proposal, and later Hagar does indeed bear him a son, Ishmael. But the plan Sarai hatched wasn't quite in keeping with the terms of the promise the Lord had made with Abram. It was an unfaithful circumvention. The urgency of having an heir seemed to justify disregard of the promise.

And as it happens, circumventing the terms of the promise carries troubling consequences. Hagar looks on Sarai with contempt, and when Sarai identifies the new scorn from her servant, she (with Abram's permission) deals harshly with her. The whole surrogacy idea was a huge mistake. God shows mercy to Hagar and Ishmael, but the child God promised through Sarai would not come for another thirteen years, by which point Abram and Sarai are so old that God's gentle reminder of his covenant, especially the promise of a child, is met with laughter. Always ready to relish good irony, God notifies them of the child's name: Isaac. Their promised son would forever bear the name of their response—*laughter.*

God delivers on his promise in his own time, not Abraham and Sarah's. Elaborate attempts to adjust the terms of God's promise were futile. In fact, their strategies were evidence of infidelity and hopelessness. Laughter was proof that they had given up hope in the promise of a child long ago. Realities of their situation were far, far too contravening. When a child finally is conceived, however, there is no question why and how it has happened: God has done it. Isaac is God's gift, the longed-for and long-awaited child of the covenant. God redeems the error of using Hagar as a surrogate, but the promise of a child was clear and his faithfulness to it was sure.

Jacob, Leah, and Rachel (Genesis 28–30). Jacob worked twice as many years as he thought he'd have to in order to wed Rachel. Laban got the best of him. Jacob thought he slept with Rachel, the one he'd worked seven years for, when really it was Leah. The trickster got tricked! He deceived his father to steal the blessing meant for his older brother, Esau, and, now on the run and under very different circumstances, he himself is deceived into marrying the wrong woman. Eventually Jacob and Laban reach an agreement and Jacob will also wed Rachel—for real this time—in return for another seven years' labor.

Jacob loves Rachel more than Leah, and because Leah is unpreferred, God "opens her womb," while Rachel remains barren (Gen. 29:31). Leah conceives many sons. Rachel none. Rachel envies her sister and dismays. She blames her plight initially on Jacob: "Give me children, or I shall die!" (Gen. 30:1). She's promptly rebuked for it. "Am I in the place of God," asks Jacob, "who has withheld from you the fruit of the womb?" (30:2). Rachel improvises. She adopts the Sarah strategy and offers Jacob her servant, who, over ensuing years, bears him two children. Meanwhile Leah, who thought her childbearing years were behind her, suddenly conceives yet another child, followed again by two more. She has seven children in all.

Leah's story is exquisitely redemptive. She is eldest but grows up in the shadow of her more dazzling sister. Her father uses her to exploit an advantage over Jacob. She knows that Jacob is enraged by this deceit and understands that she will always be for him a reminder of it. She recognizes that Rachel is Jacob's first love. She believes she is hated. Her situation can be described only as one of isolation and despair and futility. She sees only one option for carving out a meaningful existence—to bear Jacob children.

The names Leah bestows upon each of her first four sons tell us everything we need to know about her brokenness and redemption. The first she names Reuben: "Because the LORD has looked upon my affliction; for now my husband will love me." Her second she names Simeon: "Because the LORD has heard that I am hated, he has given me this son also." The third is named Levi, for "this time my husband will be attached to me, because I have borne him three sons." Leah's deepest longing is to be loved by Jacob, and she is convinced that bearing him sons will win his adoration. Her desperation is agonizing (Gen. 29:32–34).

At some point between the birth of her third and fourth son, however, Leah's heart goes through a transformation. She bestows upon her fourth son the name Judah, for "this time I will praise *the LORD*" (Gen. 29:35). The child's very name is praise. She no longer labors in vain for the affection and approval of Jacob. No longer is her value found in giving Jacob what she thinks he most wants. With the arrival of Judah she *praises God* for giving life. Unbeknownst to her, many centuries later, the very Son of God would be born in the line of this son, Judah.

"Then God remembered Rachel, and God listened to her and opened her womb" (Gen. 30:22). God extends mercy to Rachel. He makes possible what before was impossible. That imagery of "opening the womb" is wonderfully vivid. He creates the conditions for conception, for life, and almost immediately Rachel conceives. She names her son Joseph, a name that both acknowledges God's gift and requests another at the same time. Joseph's arrival is fully God's doing. He has done it. He has given life.

Elkanah and Hannah (1 Samuel 1). Elkanah has two wives, Peninnah and Hannah. Peninnah has children, but Hannah has no children (1 Sam. 1:2). Elkanah is a devout man and travels each year to Shiloh to offer his sacrifices to the Lord. As the story goes, Elkanah distributes portions of the sacrifice to Peninnah and to all his children, "but to Hannah he gave a double portion, because he loved her, though the LORD had closed her womb" (1:5). Peninnah views Hannah as a "rival" and would "provoke her grievously to irritate her" for her childlessness (1:6). These cruel provocations went on for years. "Therefore Hannah wept and would not eat" (1:7).

Elkanah attempts to console Hannah by asking why she is sad and does not eat, but also to manipulate her, pleading, "Am I not more to you than ten sons?" (1 Sam. 1:8). Relieving her sadness by questioning her love for him isn't the most empathetic approach, admittedly, and in the way of application it's a clear example of how *not* to respond to a woman's suffering. In any case, now desperate, Hannah turns to God: "O LORD of hosts, if you will indeed look on the affliction of your servant and remember me and not forget your servant, but will give to your servant a son, then I will give him to the LORD all the days of his life" (1:11). Eli the priest happens to see her praying, mouthing her petition silently and weeping in lament, and once he's convinced she's not drunk, he blesses her: "Go in peace, and the God of Israel grant your petition" (1:17).

Soon after this encounter, Hannah conceives. She names her son Samuel, because "I have asked for him from the LORD," and the Lord has heard (1 Sam. 1:20). Once the child is weaned, she dedicates him to the Lord just as she promised she would: "For this child I prayed, and the LORD has granted me my petition that I made to him. Therefore I have lent him to the LORD. As long as he lives, he is lent to the LORD" (1:27).

Hannah acknowledges that Samuel is a gift from God. Her womb was closed but "the LORD remembered her" (1 Sam. 1:19), and suddenly she is fertile. She gladly consecrates the child to God's service. Samuel bears the name of what God did.

May we pause here briefly and acknowledge the fundamental importance placed on naming children throughout the Bible? We've considered only three narratives so far, and already we notice these mothers bestow upon their children names either chosen for them by God or self-selected names reflecting God's grace and favor. Different names for different reasons, of course, but always the names are deeply meaningful and declare something about the Lord's work. He is good. He is the Giver of life. Naming children is a gesture both of thanksgiving and of hope.

Zechariah and Elizabeth (Luke 1:5–25). The final story we'll explore is from the New Testament. Zechariah is a priest. He and Elizabeth are described as "righteous before God" and "walking blamelessly in all the commandments and statutes" (Luke 1:6). But despite their righteousness they have no child, "because Elizabeth was barren, and both were advanced in years" (v. 7). There seems to be some sort of implied tension between the righteousness of the couple and their childlessness, a common theme in these narratives of infertility. But we'll come back to that momentarily.

Zechariah has the responsibility to burn incense in the temple while the people of Israel pray outside. One day, an angel visits Zechariah when he is officiating at the altar. He's told that his prayers have been heard and that Elizabeth will bear a son, whom they should name John, meaning (roughly) the "Lord is gracious." The angel informs Zechariah of what his son will do and of how God will use him. But Zechariah is skeptical. "How could I know this will happen?" he asks. "My wife and I are old."

In response the angel identifies himself as Gabriel and silences Zechariah, explaining that he will remain mute until the promised child is born. Zechariah is in the temple so long and his behavior on exit is so erratic that the people of Israel assume he's received some mystical vision from the Lord. Indeed he has, although not the kind anyone would ever have expected! Elizabeth soon conceives precisely as promised, and she thanks God for looking upon her and taking away her reproach. Conceiving a child is for her a relief from affliction.

Barren is such a blunt, searing term. It summons images of scorched and rainless earth, cracked up by the sheer absence of vitality. When applied to a woman's womb, the term connotes an austere incapacity for life. Deadness. Life does not proceed from the womb because the womb itself is lifeless. The rough synonym for the term today is *infertile*: not necessarily *incapable* of fostering life but nevertheless physiologically unaccommodating. The terms reflect their periods of use, obviously, but it's worth pointing out that whether we call it barrenness or infertility, neither presents a challenge to God. He is the Giver of life.

A word of caution is needed here on drawing too direct a connection between these infertility narratives in Genesis and infertility in the twenty-first century. God may quite suddenly open a closed womb today. Stories abound of infertile couples defying all prognoses and conceiving a child, to the shock of their physicians. Still, in our time God has providentially furnished medical means of opening wombs, means that did not exist in the ancient world. Infertility is treatable. We'll need to assess precisely which treatments are rightful expressions of God's providence at a later point in this book. For now it is enough simply to caution against the generalization that somehow God and medicine, particularly infertility treatment, are in competition.

Gospel and Childlessness

Remember again the truth of the gospel: the God who breathes creation itself into being has in Christ reaffirmed creation, and *in him is life*. He infused what he made with life and he continues to do so. His creation is not a one-time event, but is ongoing. God loves life. He's a Redeemer.

When, for example, Jesus tells Nicodemus that he must be reborn, Nicodemus takes him literally (John 3). What do you mean *reborn*? Jesus makes clear to Nicodemus that rebirth is God's doing, and refers to radically new life that the believer receives from God. Nothing is ever the same. Even the conditions of life itself are turned on their heads. In fact, Jesus goes so far as to call himself the way, truth, and *life* (John 14:6). In him is life, *and that life was the light of men* (John 1:4)!

Recalling the Genesis narratives, then, notice the clear distinction between how several of the men and women above interpret their fertility or barrenness, and what God is at the same time *doing among and through* them. Bearing children is seen as a sign of favor, of blessing. Inability to conceive and bear children is perceived as a judgment. In some cases the experience becomes a source of bitter conflict. A mother is believed somehow superior to the childless woman. But these all-too-human perceptions do not always correspond with the way God himself sees our circumstances.

Take Leah and Rachel as an example. Leah interprets her motherhood as a sort of talent and attempts to use it as a way to earn her husband's love and favor. She even antagonizes her sister with it. But God's reasons for blessing Leah with children is his *own* deciding and has nothing to do with Leah's biological or moral status. The same goes for Rachel. She has committed no obvious wrong to garner God's judgment. Her childlessness is not a punishment. When she does conceive, it is in *God's* good timing. He is with the house of Jacob and at work among them. But in saying as much, let me offer a few qualifications.

Each of the narratives we've surveyed end happily with the arrival of a long-expected child. They conclude this way for crucial theological reasons. Infertility is thematic in Genesis because God's covenant with Abraham and his descendants is in a rather overt way contingent upon *having children* whom the covenant can pass along to. If, for example, Abraham and Sarah do not have a child, then the promise God has made to Abraham is unmade. God's turning infertility into fecundity in each of these instances is a sign of his *covenant faithfulness*, of his unflagging commitment to his people. Elizabeth's conception in Luke 1 is similarly covenantal, only in this case the promised child is consecrated for the prophetic task of preparing the way for the Lord Jesus Christ. In it we are meant to detect a glimmer of what God did in Genesis.

The purpose of these narratives is not to demonstrate why and how our fruitful God always triumphs over infertility, opening what is closed and answering every petition. That is an understandable but misleading conclusion to draw. The purpose, rather, is to highlight God's covenant faithfulness. He always upholds his side of the promise.

God's promise to you and me, as members of the new covenant, as ones who have been grafted in through Christ's atoning death and victorious resurrection, is eternal life in him. Inclusion within the old covenant depended, by and large, on being born into the house of Israel. Inclusion in the new covenant, however, depends upon the redemptive grace of Jesus Christ that saves sinners. God's covenant with us in Christ transcends the former limitations of conception and lineage, adopting all who trust in him.

The new covenant is unthreatened by infertility. Under the new covenant the promise underscores *spiritual* birth, of living and preaching the gospel. The infertile are in this case the spiritually infertile, those who do not contribute to the mission of making disciples of all the nations. Infertile are those who, irrespective of how many children they may have, parent no spiritual children, point none to Christ, and rear no one to maturity. This idea may not console the biologically infertile. I impress the point on the hope that even biological infertility would be interpreted in light of Christ's kingdom and mission.

Here's what all this means for you, Christian: God may use you to advance his mission *as he so chooses*. In giving your life over to him in discipleship, you acknowledged your total dependency and thus placed yourself fully at his disposal. We cannot place exceptions or stipulations on discipleship. To paraphrase the great German theologian Dietrich Bonhoeffer, when Jesus calls a person he *bids him come and die*.[2] Earthen vessels are valuable for what they carry. The relevance of such truth to the experience of infertility is clear—how disciples will participate in God's mission, including how they will do so as part of a family, is God's determination.

Children are not an entitlement or reward, after all, but a gift. On the Christian theological account, the disciple crucified with Christ is entitled to nothing and earns nothing. To Christ all is owed. Everything the disciple has—*everything*—is received as a gift of grace. This beneficence includes bearing and rearing children. Everywhere the Scriptures reaffirm this truth. No one has a "right" to children. Whether children will be given is shrouded in sovereign mystery, calling to mind the hard but consoling words of Job: "The LORD gave, and the LORD has taken away; blessed be the name of the LORD" (Job 1:21).

In this respect one cannot help but notice that the climax in each of the fertility narratives is the birth of a long-desired child. They all have "happy" endings. As I have already remarked, the purpose in rehearsing these stories is *not* to promise childless couples the birth of their own child if they will but wait and pray and believe. That would be insensitive and perhaps even impudent advice to offer, and I think also a reckless conclusion to draw. For some couples God may provide a child of their own progeny, and for others he may not. But to all those Christian couples who have not conceived, and who may never conceive, please take the following to heart: you are not being punished, you are not comparably less faithful, you are not failures, and your prayers are not somehow less efficacious. You are God's child. You are a part of his family.

Childlessness is difficult to understand sometimes, but it is not a punitive judgment. God is himself a Father. He made the family. He loves the family. God cares for his children and hears their prayers. If you are without children, please know that God has not forgotten or forsaken you, but has instead, perhaps only for a time, *given you a slightly different way of being family and thus of participating in his life and mission.*

Takeaways

- The language of "responsibility" is inadequate to establish grounds for procreation. Under the new covenant, procreation is good because of other, higher goods God has commanded and wants for his children.
- There are some good reasons for a couple not to procreate.
- Children are not an entitlement or a reward, but a gift.
- Infertility narratives in Scripture are not implicit promises of children, but are evidence of God's commitment to his covenant and care for his children.
- God's reasons for withholding children remain a mystery to us.
- Couples may nevertheless understand infertility as God's offering a slightly different way of being family and thus of participating in his life and mission.

2

Christian Discipleship and Human Affection

John and Lizzy were still weighing their options and contemplating IVF when, one bright summer afternoon, a home pregnancy test returned positive. Lizzy couldn't—*wouldn't*—believe it. Display of that plus sign after so many years of negatives struck her as cruelly implausible. She hid the test in a medicine cabinet and decided to try another test the following morning. The first one might be mistaken.

Sleep eluded her that night. In that dark, quiet stillness she prayed with a hopeful furor, mouthing pleas and spilling tears until empty before God. Exhausted, a dreamless sleep finally overtook her.

It took several licks across the face from their hound to rouse Lizzy the following morning. She could barely open her eyes, they were so swollen. Scratching the dog's head she swung out of bed and stumbled into the kitchen for coffee. She told herself she would finish the first cup and dress for the day before trying another pregnancy test. Two short sips and a daydream later she found herself magically in the bathroom gazing at another equally magical plus sign. With a giddy smile she sprinted to her room, threw on the first clothes she could find, and raced out the door for John's office.

John was examining blueprints when Lizzy burst into his office effusive, puffy, and unkempt. He straightened and gazed at her open-mouthed, summoning every sense organ to reorient himself to the moment. The excitement that propelled Lizzy through the office door accelerated the closer she approached John. Throwing her arms around his neck without slowing nearly tumbled them both to the floor. John laughed loud at the incongruity of it all. Upright and balanced again, Lizzy produced from her pocket the positive pregnancy test, explaining what John saw with his eyes in case, like her, his first response was disbelief. He took the rest of the day off.

Several weeks later Lizzy shifted nervously on the ultrasound examination table, its thin medical paper crinkling underneath her. John would have paced if the room hadn't been so small. Both of them directed their nervousness unconsciously toward the smiling ultrasound tech the moment she entered the room. Something in the confidence of her smile suggested she was experienced, a perception confirmed by her efficient command of the equipment. Pleasantries and humor also helped.

Initial images appearing on the monitor mounted to the wall were indecipherable. They peered unblinking at the screen. To their mutual surprise the first affirmation they had longed for wasn't produced visibly, but audibly, and caught them by complete surprise—a *heartbeat*! A heartbeat so unmistakable, so human, so rapid and urgent they reached for each other's hand partly out of affection and partly to ground each other in the astonishing levity of the moment.

Ultrasound photos promptly appeared on the refrigerator. As John and Lizzy approached the second trimester, they jubilantly announced the news to parents, family, and close friends. John and Lizzy remarked often to each other on how surreal it all felt; having dreamed of having a child for so long, they initially found the *reality* of pregnancy hard to accept. But they quickly adjusted to the new normal. Lizzy's morning sickness was a daily reminder, and John never tired of late-night jaunts to pick up Lizzy's newest craving. They'd settled into something of a routine.

Inexplicably, shortly after returning home from lunch with friends one Tuesday, Lizzy miscarried. As suddenly as the pregnancy was discovered, it was lost. Lizzy was inconsolable. John did what John usually did in moments of volatility, which was to slip into the role of resolute stoic, steady but emotionally detached. He told himself that what Lizzy most needed was constancy and evenness. They both told themselves lots of things as they adjusted to a child not coming.

Through it all, from the first giddy days of pregnancy to that desolate Tuesday, John and Lizzy clung to God in dependency and hope. They doubted God, of course, especially at the beginning. What redemptive or providential reason could possibly justify the death of their little one? They were grieving. Time is what they needed, and with each passing week they were reminded gradually of God's kindness. He was their Lord before they ever conceived, just as he was their Lord in the midst of loss. They were *disciples*, after all—where else could they turn?

Where We're Going

That question—*Where else could they turn?*—is an instructive one. The Bible describes disciples of Jesus Christ as sojourners, as people who learn from him how to live *with* him and advance his mission. Discipleship makes sense of who we fundamentally are in Christ. When the rug is pulled out from under us, when crisis upends all our givens, the disciple not only looks to Jesus for bearings, but clings *to* him and pleads *with* him and learns *from* him.

The purpose of this chapter is to outline some of the basic theological truths of Christian discipleship and to apply these truths to the experience of infertility. Hopefully it reviews some of what you already understand about discipleship, and if so, I'd ask that you stick with it, because I also want to address a comparably neglected power of discipleship: human affection.

We are *desiring* creatures. We want things. And these affections have astonishing power over us. This is especially true when we are at a "where to turn?" point in life, because it is at precisely this point that we glimpse the true character of our own discipleship. When hurled into some dark and threatening vortex, is our answer to the question human, earthly, and carnal, or is it instead a simple admission: "I believe; help my unbelief!" (Mark 9:24).

The Nature of Discipleship

Discipleship is a theological concept that deserves our careful attention. It is central to the story of Jesus's ministry. From the beginning he calls sinners, hypocrites, and outcasts to enter discipleship with him, and those who follow are forever changed. The same is true for us. In discipleship our lives are fundamentally redefined by our relationship with Christ Jesus.

46

When Jesus explains this transformative change in human personality to Nicodemus, he uses the vivid imagery of rebirth (John 3). Discipleship with Jesus Christ is like starting life over, but on entirely different terms and with an entirely different purpose. A believer *is* a disciple. Our whole lives are reoriented to Jesus Christ. Even if we know what discipleship means and involves, it is nevertheless important to remember its profound reshaping of our beliefs, feelings, and actions. Our very agency is rescued and vindicated.

Discipleship isn't just a concept. It is a reality-defining relationship. The moment we ask about the "hows" of discipleship—"How do we become one with Christ?" and "How are we to live as one with Christ?"—we are at once confronted with the mercy and goodness and power and wisdom and majesty of Jesus Christ. Jesus calls, Jesus redeems, Jesus admonishes, Jesus leads, and Jesus sends. *He* sets the terms of discipleship. *He* is the good teacher.

Our individual testimonies of Christ's redemption resemble those of Jesus's first disciples. In Matthew 4:18–20, for example, Jesus is walking beside the Sea of Galilee and spots a couple of brothers fishing. He calls out to Peter and Andrew: "Follow me, and I will make you fishers of men" (v. 19). The text includes no gap or ellipsis or pause; the brothers immediately leave their nets to follow him. Our own answer to the question of how do we become disciples resembles that of Peter and Andrew: Christ comes to us, calls us, and then teaches us how to live with and for him.

Christ comes to us. We could not in our sin go to him. He alone is the Mediator between God and man. He is our reconciliation. And when Jesus comes to us, he calls. This call is not simply a wistful, open-ended invitation. Christ's call is also a command: *follow me*. He is to be believed and he is to be obeyed. In discipleship, faith and obedience are inseparable. Christ both invites and commands relationship with him. For Peter and Andrew this relationship appeared on first glance as simply one between student and teacher, but discipleship is a great deal more than that. Much more.[1]

Disciples learn gradually over time the fuller implications of this call to learn at Jesus's side. It is, despite its obvious simplicity, also a mysterious and paradoxical call. Jesus's call is a call to life through *death*. That is how the apostle Paul understood it. The disciple of Jesus is crucified with him, so that it is no longer the disciple who lives, but Christ that lives within him (Gal. 2:20). Being a disciple doesn't just involve death to self in wholehearted allegiance to Christ, but requires it. The disciple is a dead person whose only life is Christ. As the great German theologian Dietrich Bonhoeffer so memorably put it, "When Christ calls a man, he bids him come and die!"[2] In this death we find eternal life!

Discipleship consists in faith *and* obedience. Our faith has a genuine first moment, and is also ongoing. This faith is not, however, self-generating. Rather faith comes from hearing, and hearing through the Word of God (Rom. 10:17). We believe Christ only because Christ addresses us. He pronounces the word we most need to hear—the word of redemption in Christ—and enables us to hear it as it must be heard. That word, again, may for us have a first hearing, yet it is reproclaimed again and again, such that the disciple would do well to heed the counsel of James and "put away all filthiness and rampant wickedness and receive with meekness the implanted word, which is able to save your souls" (James 1:21). We believe and are then commanded and encouraged to keep on believing.

The Greek term for *obedience* in the New Testament, *hypakoē*, which translates "beneath the word," also applies to hearing Jesus. We get our modern English term *acoustics* from the root, *akoe*, or "hearing." In this linguistic context, obedience represents one's willingness to hear, acknowledge, and submit to an authority. Disciples obey what they hear because of where, or from whom, the word comes (or from where it originates), not because of some abstract rule or principle. Discipleship is a personal relationship with Christ.

A prerequisite to obeying the Word of God is hearing the Word of God. Not "hearing" in our purely auditory sense, but in the deeper spiritual sense captured by Christ when he commands anyone with ears to hear, "let him hear." Jesus says, "My sheep hear my voice, and I know them, and they follow me" (John 10:27). Sheep hear the voice of their shepherd, who knows them, and in hearing the shepherd's voice they follow him. It is a familiar, welcome voice. In this sense, hearing and obedience are coterminous. To hear the shepherd is all the sheep need to follow him.

The life of discipleship is also a life of learning. A disciple is an intimate student of Jesus Christ. Jesus has already cleansed the disciple in his own righteousness, and now through the power of the Spirit he enables the disciple to learn at his side. Genuine learners accept that they are not already in possession of all wisdom. Disciples recognize that wisdom comes from Christ, or "from above," as James puts. The difference between heavenly and earthly wisdom is displayed fundamentally in the fruit yielded in one's life. Earthly wisdom is jealous and self-seeking, whereas wisdom from above is "first pure, then peaceable, gentle, open to reason, full of mercy and good fruits, impartial and sincere" (James 3:17). Wisdom that comes from Christ is therefore self-effacing and sacrificial, answering the question posed by James (v. 13)—"Who is wise and understanding among you?"—with a simple answer: those eager to receive *Christ's* wisdom.

Salvation is a gift. No one deserves or earns a relationship with God. He comes to us; he calls us; he teaches us to live with him and for him. It is a gift extended to us in mercy and thus received with gratitude. We are perhaps sometimes tempted to think of our standing with God as some tacit entitlement to expect great personal advantages. It is, after all, the relationship with maximal, even everlasting benefits. But that belief, that impulse, is a *temptation*, one James memorably portrays in the first chapter of his epistle: "Each person is tempted when he is lured and enticed by his own desire" (James 1:14). We are tempted to think we have some sort of claim on Jesus.

In truth, the only rightful way to understand discipleship is to accept that Christ has full and exclusive claim upon his disciples. That is because he is not merely our teacher; he is our Lord. He created us by his breath and redeems us by his blood. The Son of God gave his very life. Reconciliation is therefore entirely his to offer. And so we stand as wretched, undeserving recipients of his loving-kindness, for "every good gift and every perfect gift is from above, coming down from the Father of lights, with whom there is no variation or shadow due to change" (James 1:17).

Grace is a gift no one can afford to buy or afford to refuse. If, then, the grace of God is a gift, and if we have no claim upon Christ but he has every claim upon us, then whatever goods we receive from God should be received in a spirit of gratitude and deference. We are in his eternal debt and depend wholly upon his favor.

The fact that children are a gift from the Lord is a hard truth for parents and childless alike (Ps. 127:3). The truth is hard in different ways, naturally, but nevertheless demands similar affirmation. No couple is entitled to children. Precisely because children are a gift and not an entitlement, we should understand having or not having children as part of God's purposes for us as disciples on mission with him. With or without children, disciples are commissioned to live and proclaim the good news of Jesus Christ. Those missions may have a different shape or focus or approach, yet still configure into Christ's grand mission of making disciples. Every disciple of Jesus Christ is *first* a disciple, and then, in light of that first-order relation, he or she occupies other roles.

This is why I say that *the Creator and Redeemer of life has not forsaken the infertile but has instead given them a slightly different way of being family and thus of participating in the life and mission of God.* Every child of God has a calling. A calling is not simply to a job or profession, although that it is how the term is commonly applied. A calling applies to a particular way God invites us to live in the world. One may be called to the law or to the classroom, to singleness or to marriage (1 Corinthians 7), to child-rearing or to childlessness. The call—and reasons for it—are Christ's alone.

Affections

Humans are both thinking and feeling creatures. Our beliefs are always accompanied by feelings, and our feelings are always accompanied by our beliefs. Humans have *affections*, and our affections propel us toward action. Affections fuel action. We act, in part, to satisfy desire.

We all have needs and wants, and to some extent we all understand that needs and wants are distinguishable. I need coffee each morning but I don't really need a million dollars. I need decent shelter when tornado season cycles through Oklahoma each year, but I don't need a Florentine estate (nice as it would be to vacation at one). A caffeine fix, a shelter from a storm—these are sensibly called needs. A million big ones and a Florentine estate can only be described as wants.

The problem isn't that we don't see the distinction between needs and wants, but that we live as though the distinction is collapsible. Our talent for elevating a want to a need is limitless. We acquire some new thing or have some new experience, develop a fondness for it, and almost instantly that thing or experience morphs from a want into a need. Did you notice that I described coffee as a need, even though it's really a want? My heavy addiction isn't enough to justify reclassifying it, and this is only one, somewhat superficial, example. We refer to all sorts of things as needs that are not really needs, strictly speaking, but are things we've developed dependencies for.

It goes without saying that the more dependent we are on something, the less we are able to do without it. Obvious as it is, however, we nevertheless find it difficult both to *identify* when we have formed a new dependency and to *acknowledge* the depth of our enduring dependencies. Now, this in itself isn't a problem. Dependencies are something we all have. Disciples are of necessity dependent upon Jesus Christ, and the church is by definition an interdependent people, a community eager to give and receive gifts from one another. Dependency becomes a problem when the object depended upon is corrupt or degrading. A sure sign that an object is corrupt or degrading is its direct malformation of human personality. Things we shouldn't be dependent upon change us for the worse. One word we use to describe this sort of alteration is *addiction*.

Occasionally, through a series of gradual and unacknowledged assumptions, we can even come to see a thing as something we deserve. Up to this point I've been talking about our wants and needs relative to this abstract noun, "things." But if you think about it, sometimes we assume children are somehow deserved. We're human, after all, and so it's natural to think of having children as requisite to the marital relationship. The main impetus to this assumption is its opposite. We think of children as the familial norm, and so consider it unfair *not* to be able to have children. Articulating our specific reasons for these assumptions isn't something we're especially good at.

Scripture is clear that children are not something couples are entitled to. Each and every child is a gift. No one is entitled to a gift. It is possible to become angry at the unfairness of not receiving the gift of children, just as it is possible to feel it unfair not to have a "normal" experience like having children. But let me ask: what is normal about Christianity? Ours is a strange faith. Endlessly peculiar. Bizarre even. It challenges norms and establishes its own. The norm in Christianity is the person of Jesus Christ. Because he is the norm, his revelation is normative. He sets the standard. His commands *must* be obeyed. Just think here of his stunning words in the Sermon on the Mount: "You have heard that it was said. . . . But I say to you" (Matthew 5–7). He challenges even our most settled notions of what counts as normalcy.

It is easy to conflate our own privileged, conventional norms with distinctly Christian norms. We are pathologically presumptuous creatures. Yet, part of what it means to be sanctified by the Holy Spirit is to have one's commitments and affections brought into accord with God's purposes. "Present your bodies as a living sacrifice," exhorts Paul. "Do not be conformed to this world, but be transformed by the renewal of your mind" (Rom. 12:1–2). Discipleship consists of learning from God how to live for God, which includes the renewal of our commitments and affections.

God calls disciples to participate in his ongoing mission. Our callings are not strictly labor-related, as I've said, but they also involve marriage and singleness. In 1 Corinthians 7 Paul responds to a question regarding the shape of Christian marriage by explaining, among other things, why the unmarried may wisely remain unmarried, under what conditions the unmarried should marry, why married couples of different faiths may remain married, and even why widows should remain unmarried. It gets pretty detailed. By the end of his assessment, Paul makes clear that Christians can be called of God to marriage *or* to singleness. "I wish that all were as I myself am," he admits. "But each has his own gift from God, one of one kind and one of another" (1 Cor. 7:7). Some can and should marry, while others can and should remain single. Both are legitimate and important callings.

Author Karen Swallow Prior has suggested that it is possible to understand childlessness, too, as a calling.[3] The idea isn't expressly commended in 1 Corinthians 7, nor does it appear in other epistles. Yet, difficult as this idea "childlessness as calling" may be for some, it is nevertheless a fruitful way of understanding infertility. Just as the single person can participate in God's mission differently from the married person, so too can the childless couple participate differently in God's mission than couples with children. Thinking of childlessness not as a reproach but as a calling frees disciples to discern how they are to participate in God's mission on the terms God has set.

Accepting this truth is difficult precisely because of our affections. Yearning for a long-awaited child may prompt a range of emotions, including anger, rage, despair, bitterness, and resentment. These are natural affective responses anyone may harbor toward God when it seems God is not furnishing children he just as well could furnish. From our limited human point of view, God's withholding strikes us as arbitrary, and arbitrariness fosters resentment. But God's withholding is never arbitrary, even when it involves children. Acknowledging this truth—acknowledging God's kindness and faithfulness—is essential to tempering the emotional tumult of infertility. Childlessness is not punitive, it is not arbitrary, and it is not wrong. It is—troubling as it may be to accept—a kind of calling.

None of this implies that a couple may not continue to want and pray for a child of their own. I am not in any way commending resignation. It is entirely possible to rest fully in God's contentment, to affirm his purposes, and to accept his will, and at the same time to implore him ardently for children.

The essence of prayer is request. Prayer is affective. Always. Our prayers are saturated with feelings. We have a need or want, and petition God for help. This isn't defiance: it's faithfulness. And we hope for a resolute confidence like Paul's—to learn that in whatever situation, we are "to be content" (Phil. 4:11). This is as true for couples only beginning to be concerned about their infertility as it is for couples who have long since accepted the childlessness that infertility imposed upon them.

Contentment is resting in the grace and sufficiency of God. It's not luxuriant recline in decadent excess, or a life unencumbered by difficulty or hardship. When the Epistles encourage Christians to be content, they often do so in the context of scarcity. Because disciples are always to think of their lives as "for Christ's sake," they are to mimic the apostle Paul and become "content with weaknesses, insults, hardships, persecutions, and calamities" (2 Cor. 12:10). Contentment always implies surrender and trust: a surrender of the self to God and trust in God's abundant grace. God alone is the source of all true and lasting contentment.

Good News for God's People

Christ's disciples are as variegated and eclectic a crew as you can imagine. He draws his church from all corners of the earth. He saves all types. The relationship he offers us with him is pure in two senses: pure in that he in his perfect righteousness is our atonement and reconciliation with God, and pure also in that discipleship precludes exceptions or conditions. When we attempt to insert an adjective to qualify the kind of disciple we are, we have at once erred. I am not a "white" Christian or a "straight" Christian or even an "American" Christian. I am simply a Christian—by God's grace—and all other identities are interpreted in light of that reality. I am first a Christian who *happens* to have other associative roles. All that I am is subject to Christ. The same goes for all Christ's disciples, for all who have been crucified with him (Gal. 2:20) and whose lives are hidden with Christ in God (Col. 3:3). We are most who we are *because* of him, *in* him.

Do we sometimes place qualifications on discipleship when it comes to children? Unquestionably. We harbor tacit expectations about the exact shape our discipleship should take. These expectations often function as controls we wish to place on our futures, to fix the plot points of our stories and coordinate the specifics of our destiny. We look on our respective horizons and, if we're honest, we simply want Jesus to come alongside whatever it is we want to do. Things need to go the way we've already decided they should go, including a dreamed-of family.

Jesus's call to discipleship inverts all that. He puts a question to our certainties and pretenses. Isn't that part of what's going on when God commands Abraham to sacrifice his son Isaac? Abraham relishes the fruit of God's promise, relaxes in the knowledge of its certainty, until, quite suddenly, everything is threatened; the son of promise is to be slain by his own father (Genesis 22). That story illustrates a great many things, but one of its truths relevant to parenting and childlessness is this: children are received as a gift *from* God to be reared in faith *for* God. The command to Abraham is all the evidence we need that Isaac was always God's child. Abraham's obedience is all the evidence we need that he grasped the authority and power of God.

Our penchant for placing conditions on how God *must* use us in the mission he has called us to is one of the more glaring indicators of disbelief in the Christian life. We somehow become committed to a future of our own desiring and construction, rather than to what seems an unpredictable, even risky adventure with Jesus. We think we know better than God what he needs from us. It is a crafty, recurring lie we tell ourselves. As Jesus reminds us in his Sermon, no one can serve two masters (Matt. 6:24).

This same lie is at the root of all the mistaken identities we assume. We don't just want to possess and achieve certain things for ourselves, we want *others to see us* possess and achieve certain things for ourselves. Optics are a personal priority. We devise elaborate strategies for protecting and projecting our image. We dread embarrassment and delight in accolades. And yet, if we are honest with ourselves, we recognize the superficiality of our antics and perhaps even feel the Spirit's conviction.

What we're doing is trying to find our identity in something or someone other than God. Even parenthood can become a form of identity-seeking, possibly with a desire for children exceeding the desire for God. Or, similarly, a parent can turn children into a project of self-fulfillment, and neglect the responsibility to point children to Christ and to help form them in wisdom and love. Parenthood, too, can become an idol.

Whether or not we have children of our own, discipleship enables us to understand our place in the world. Jesus invites us to life with him, and in following him we accept that he sets the terms of our existence. There's no such thing as discipleship without surrender. In this surrender, paradoxically, our agency is fully realized. We are *Christ's*. We are his children—sons and daughters of the Most High. He is our King. We are employees or employers, teachers or students, buyers or sellers, runners or bikers, elders or deacons, defenders or prosecutors, parents or children *as* disciples of Jesus Christ. A disciple is *how* we are those things.

For infertile readers, my purpose in expounding at length on discipleship and human affection is to remind you that following Christ is not merely a matter of acknowledging his authority, but of being content in his authority. Contentment implies zealous excitement for God on the move, a readiness to put oneself at his disposal, a hope in his kingdom at hand. Contentment requires deep, prolonged formation in the Holy Spirit. Contentment is learned by abiding in him and dwelling with him. It is one of his fruits. We learn what it means to have children, or not to have children, as children of the One who made us and redeemed us, and who keeps us to the end.

Takeaways

- Christian discipleship implies—indeed requires—death to self.
- All ends and purposes a disciple may have are subordinate to Jesus Christ.
- Discipleship is about hearing, believing, and obeying the Word of God.
- Even parenthood, or desire to be a parent, is subject to Jesus and his mission.
- A result of following Jesus should be that we desire what Christ desires.
- We must be prepared to repent of desires held too firmly or which cause us either to ignore or reject Jesus's purposes for us.
- We must repent of conditions or stipulations we place on how or when we are Christ's disciples.
- The only sure place to find identity is in Jesus Christ.
- Contentment and perseverance come from the Holy Spirit of God.

3

The Vitality and Consolation
of the Church

The same family and friends who celebrated with John and Lizzy in those early weeks of pregnancy now, following the miscarriage, rallied to them with compassion and generosity. Lizzy descended into melancholy and was frequently overwhelmed by fits of sobbing. John had never seen her like this. He held her shaking body and absorbed her mournful tears and whispered the same thing he told himself: *it's ok*. Everything slowed for her. She slept late and retired early, rarely changing out of her pajamas. She showered until the hot water turned cold. For the first two weeks following the miscarriage she lived in the bed or on the couch. Her life was about emotional survival.

John didn't do much more than hold Lizzy and be physically present to her, because he didn't really know what to do with himself. He felt as though cold winds gusted through his insides. Circles developed under his youthful eyes. He took the dog on abnormally long walks. He assumed all cooking responsibilities. Several unfinished yard projects were promptly completed, as he threw himself into anything that would distract him from despondency. And he wept, although not around Lizzy.

The fog of lament was somehow less thick and suffocating when friends and family dropped by. Lizzy's folks were especially scrupulous in their caretaking. Words were few, yet Lizzy marveled many months later as she reflected upon how discerning and sacrificial her parents had been during that anguished season. They seemed to know exactly what to do and what not to do.

John and Lizzy felt similar gratitude for their pastors and church community group. Pastors came not with platitudes or naïve promises that another child would someday come along, but with a listening silence and gentle presence. They simply affirmed the pain by sitting with John and Lizzy and crying with them. When finally they spoke, it was to console. "Man, that's hard." "I'm so, so sorry this happened to you." "We made extra for dinner and thought you could use a meal." They were prayed with and they were prayed for.

It was well over a month before John and Lizzy felt up to returning to church. Up to that point they hadn't really felt the unction to return, in part because the church had come to them. When they hurt, the body hurt. They were the wound the body attended to. Still, walking through the church parking lot hand in hand, they were pensive. How would other members they hadn't seen react? What might they say? What if a baby cried during service?

John and Lizzy sang a few rote choruses but otherwise felt displaced. Song hadn't yet returned to their hearts. They sat, rejoined hands, and as the Scripture reading was announced, flipped thoughtlessly to the text: Psalm 84:1–4. They stared blankly at their Bibles, vision blurry and minds dizzied with preoccupations. The passage was read clearly and patiently for the congregation, and its effect upon John and Lizzy was like the sensation of aloe cooling scorched flesh, only inward. What began as sound quickly became a message. They recognized it as a word for them:

> How lovely is your dwelling place,
>> O LORD of hosts!
> My soul longs, yes, faints
>> for the courts of the LORD;
> my heart and flesh sing for joy
>> to the living God.
> Even the sparrow finds a home,
>> and the swallow a nest for herself,
>> where she may lay her young,
> at your altars, O LORD of hosts,
>> my King and my God.
> Blessed are those who dwell in your house,
>> ever singing your praise! (Ps. 84:1–4)

The reading concluded, and they looked upon one another knowingly, tears filling their eyes. It was a word they desperately needed to hear. They felt the Word had visited them, as though all of existence had been arranged in the time before time for them to hear it. In the weeks to come this Word would give them some purchase on their lives again. They could live again because of this Word. Years later they would continue to remark on how this one hearing of the Word served as a fixed point of orientation at a time when, in the words of the psalmist, their souls were in Sheol.

Their church had been God's gentle means of grace during those desperate weeks. Their brothers and sisters in Christ were sources of consolation and light. They finally understood in a way they hadn't before what the apostle Paul means when he characterizes the church as a *family* and as a *body*. They belonged to a people for whom membership and mission go hand in hand.

The purpose of this chapter is to explain why belonging to and serving the church matters. Disciples of Jesus aren't alone. They don't stand apart as independent or self-sustaining. To be a disciple is to be with other disciples, together following Jesus. In this way belonging implies serving. The metaphors of *family* and *body* remind us of what it really means to follow Christ and to live in community with others as though his gospel really is good news. This church is a people constituted by God's grace, and includes fertile and infertile alike.

Membership and Mission

When God sets the people of Israel apart, he does so on special terms. He is to be their God, and they will be his people (Ex. 6:7). God always keeps his promise. He is faithful to his covenant with Israel even when Israel is wayward and rebellious.[1] God makes it clear to Israel that they are who they are and have what they have (e.g., the Promised Land) only because of God's favor. The Lord determines their whole identity as a people. The distinctly modern idea of self-forged identity is foreign to them. The fact they are *his* is what most defines them.

That is what God intended, anyway. Sometimes Israel acknowledges who God is and thus who they are, and sometimes they do not. Irrespective of circumstance, whether faithful in the

Promised Land or exiled in captivity, their purpose was to worship and obey the Lord their God, and in doing so express *why* they were a people set apart in the first place. God is their maker and deliverer. As Oliver O'Donovan has put it, God is Israel's salvation, judge, and possessor. The only proper response to the Lord is praise.[2]

Israel was to be the Lord's people among the nations. They were permitted neither to seclude themselves nor to shun or neglect the foreigner. Yes, there were conflicts. Yes, there were more than a few protracted wars. Yes, they were exiled on more than one occasion. Yes, they lived up to their name as a people who "wrestle with God." Despite all the hardship, however, God had a definite purpose for Israel. He had a mission for them. They were set apart *for mission*. They were his people and as such were to make his name known to the nations. In contemporary parlance, Israel was supposed to be a *missional* people. Being God's people was their mission.

The church, established through the blood of the new covenant, shares a lingering similarity with Israel in that the church is also a people set apart by God to participate in his mission. Jesus calls each of us out, just as he called out those first disciples. That's what *ekklesia* means: the called-out ones. We are called out of sin and into his righteousness, called out of the world and into the community he has set apart in love. He does the calling, and his Spirit bonds his adopted children in unity.

As his people we live for him. The church understands itself as having been called out so as to, in a sense, go right back in again! The church is a people set apart to bear witness to the good news in Jesus Christ. As his people we are compelled by love to make known to the nations the grace and insurpassable majesty of Christ Jesus. Christians are Christ's ambassadors, his messengers, his children and friends. Making his name known is why they are set apart.

So, membership and mission go hand in hand. Disciples of Jesus belong to the church, and those who belong to the church serve the church. A member of Christ's body is by definition also someone on mission. The Bible describes the life of the church in a couple of ways: as being like a family and being like a body. Let's explore them in turn.

Church as Family

Each of us is born into a family. We don't have a say in the matter. We're born, and that's where we find ourselves. We first come to some sense of ourselves in the context of family; we understand our place in relation to others—parents, siblings, etc.—who love and care for us. It's also why we tend to think of home and family as almost equivalent: here we are placed in the world with each other. Novelist Jonathan Franzen's description of family as the "house's soul" captures the idea rather elegantly, I think.[3] We need and want family.

Even if we consider our family strange or atypical, there are some essential features of what it means to be a family that are universal. With the exception of choosing a spouse, we don't decide who is and isn't family. We're given to each other. We *belong* to a family. It's the discreet conditions of belonging that get complicated. How we came to belong, why members can become estranged, what to do when we've got nothing more to family than accidents of kinship: these are the sorts of challenges that make finding a "typical" family impossible. All families are atypical. Yours has its weirdness; mine has its weirdness.

For a variety of peculiar cultural reasons, many today find it difficult to settle on a definition of "family." We needn't get into the technicalities of that debate here. For our purposes we can simply say that "family" describes our primary relationship nexus. We think of husband and wife, parent and child, sibling and sibling as primary, perhaps as "immediate" family, while cousins or grandparents or godchildren are "extended." This means "family" can apply to a single relationship between two people, like a husband and wife or a single mother and child.

Adopted children are family. They were not born into their family but are lovingly brought into a family on the conviction and hope that family is what they'll always be to one another from then on out. They belong and have a place. The Latin origin of the word *adopt* connotes something akin to "choosing," and adoptive parents often admit to feeling like *they* were chosen for the adoption—not by the child, of course, but by God. God brought them to one another.

Being redeemed by Jesus Christ means we are adopted as his sons and daughters. When we are estranged and undeserving, Christ through his Spirit comes to us and brings us into his family: "The Spirit himself bears witness with our spirit that we are children of God, and if children, then heirs—heirs of God and fellow heirs with Christ" (Rom. 8:16–17). By him we cry out, "Abba! Father!" (8:15). Paul says something similar to the church at Galatia: now that Christ has come, we are no longer slaves, but children, heirs of the promise, Abraham's offspring (Gal. 3:25–4:7). We are adopted as sons and daughters through Jesus Christ, "according to the purpose of his will, to the praise of his glorious grace, with which he has blessed us in the Beloved" (Eph. 1:5–6).

In God's family *everyone* is adopted. God comes to us and brings us in. He is our dwelling place, as the psalmist put it so poetically (Psalm 90). We are his sons and daughters, and we are brothers and sisters to one another. As God's children we are *with* one another and *for* one another. That doesn't mean this family life will be perfect or predictable, of course. It means simply that we're in this together. We have a common endeavor. And we do well to remember that, despite our gruesome sinfulness, Christ adopted each of us for life eternal with him.

Married or single, orphaned or adopted, fertile or infertile, close or estranged: the Christian always has a family. To believe upon the Lord Jesus Christ is to belong. As his child, alongside brothers and sisters, here we learn participation in God's mission. We find ourselves *here*, not somewhere else, and *now*, not some other time. We are to discern the terms and circumstances of our lives, to interpret them, and to bear witness to the good news in Jesus Christ.

"Let each person lead the life that the Lord has assigned to him, and to which God has called him," says Paul. "This is my rule in all the churches" (1 Cor. 7:17). Such strong language! A rule for all the churches? It is clear from the text Paul means exactly what he says. He gives two instructive examples: the circumcised and the bondservant. In the case of the former, if circumcised, do not seek to remove marks of circumcision, and if uncircumcised, do not seek circumcision. For the latter, if a bondservant, do not seek to be free unless you can realistically obtain freedom, and conversely, if free, do not seek to become enslaved.

I say these are instructive because "circumcision" and "bond-service" designate two of the most basic social identifiers of the ancient world. A son born into the house of Israel is circumcised as a sign of the covenant. Circumcision=Jew. Tribe and ethnicity represent basic social identifiers. The same goes for bondservice, which functions as an indicator of socio-economic status. Even in the modern world it is difficult to locate two more basic identities than nationality and occupation.

The context for Paul's rule is marriage and singleness, but I believe the principle applies also to couples with and without children. The family is differently constituted and thus is differently called. Different challenges and opportunities present themselves, yet each has its own definite task. Living and proclaiming the gospel is not dependent upon having children of one's own. The mission is the same. Only the conditions for carrying out that mission differ, in one case single and the other married, in one case with children and the other without. This would not have been feasible under the old covenant because the promise was in some sense contingent on Israel's continued propagation. Under the new covenant, however, *spiritual rebirth* rather than natural birth brings us into God's family.

This fact of having been adopted into God's family has direct application to how we think of our own families. Family is calling. And just as singleness or marriage contributes to our respective callings, so too does parenting and childlessness. Only God knows the exact reasons for these respective callings. None of them are "easy." Yet the terms of discipleship are such that we give ourselves to God—*all* of ourselves—and receive from him what we need to live and to serve.

This doesn't mean our pain and suffering will be less acute. We expect hardships because God tells us in his Word that we should expect hardships. James goes so far as to say we should "count it all joy, my brothers, when you meet trials of various kinds, for you know that the testing of your faith produces steadfastness. And let steadfastness have its full effect, that you may be perfect and complete, lacking in nothing" (James 1:2–4). This text is easier to read than apply, admittedly; yet all who follow Christ will suffer, some in one way and some in another.

Some Christians describe themselves as "suffering" from infertility or childlessness. They describe it that way perhaps because of the fear it induces, the joys it leaves unsavored, or the wounds it leaves unmended. Couples who want to have children, and who have not been able to do so, *hurt*. That hurt is often compounded by the fact that it isn't shared. Infertile couples often keep their infertility private, to shield themselves from the gaze and judgment of others. But it is precisely at this point, in the midst of fear, embarrassment, anxiety, or shame, that couples should understand themselves as part of a family that listens, cares, and consoles. If that is you, dear reader, please know that you are not alone. You are part of a family. Acknowledging your fears and worries, speaking your experience aloud to those you trust, is part of what being a family is all about. So, ask yourself, are you allowing your brothers and sisters in Christ to *be* family to you?

Church as Body

The apostle Paul also uses a body metaphor to capture the way God's people are united in mission. In 1 Corinthians 12, for example, Paul outlines precisely how God achieves unity in the midst of diversity. There are diverse gifts, services, and activities in the faith community, yet one Spirit, Lord, and God (1 Cor.

12:4–6). Paul says, "Just as the body is one and has many members, and all the members of the body, though many, are one body, so it is with Christ" (12:12). Not many bodies, but one. Not one member, but many. Within the unity of the body *every* part is needed; no one is inessential. These members are gifted and used by God for the advance of his kingdom. This means all the members have needs they cannot meet themselves, and so rely upon other members of the body with whom they are united.

No parts of the body can say they have no need of other parts. Disciples of Jesus Christ, members of his body, are not permitted to reject the ministry of the church. Being a part of the body requires willingness to reciprocate. Members give and receive. This truth runs directly counter to prevailing modern ideals of autonomy, self-determination, and independence. The church is by definition a community of interdependence. To believe on the Lord Jesus Christ is to, at the same time, join others in that believing. Nobody's boot-strapping it in the body of Christ! Nobody is an island.

Belonging to Christ's body implies readiness to give and to receive. We don't get to hold others at arm's length, and we aren't to withhold our gifts and contributions from others. This doesn't necessarily mean, of course, that we share anything and everything about ourselves indiscriminately. Nor should we foist ourselves upon others irrespective of their needs or concerns. We are for one another in *love*. According to Augustine, human communities are united by their common objects of love.[4] Through the power of the Holy Spirit we are united in our common love of Jesus Christ, the Head of the body (Col. 1:18). We are bound together in Christ by his love.

Conclusion

Infertility is an ecclesial experience. Membership *in* Christ implies mission *with* Christ. As his redeemed we're in this together. The mutuality and reciprocity that define the church apply to both fertile and infertile alike. Infertile couples should not, and indeed cannot, fully shoulder the burdens of their experience. They need the support of others.

Abide in me, and I in you, instructs Jesus to his disciples. "Whoever abides in me and I in him, he it is that bears much fruit, for apart from me you can do nothing" (John 15:5). He goes on to explain that to abide in him is also to abide in his love. He loves his disciples. Then he says, "This is my commandment, that you love one another as I have loved you" (15:12). God intends his church to be a community of love. He commissions his witnesses to be extensions of his love. To belong to Christ's body is to participate in his love. This body is comprised of all types, no one more or less needed than others. The Greek term the church has used to refer to its own life together is *koinonia*—Christian fellowship, sharing, and communication. Togetherness! Because Christ is for us, we are inescapably and by definition for one another.

For all of these reasons it should be clear that infertile couples need the church, and the church needs infertile couples. The ability or inability to have children is not irrelevant to the mission couples have in the church, but neither is procreative capacity all-decisive. The respective experiences have their own challenges and possibilities, their own shape. The ecclesial purpose for each couple, however, remains the same: to love God, love one another, and make known the gospel. Any ability or inability to have children must be interpreted in light of the mission we're given to embody and advance. We all must preach the gospel to ourselves, and in doing so learn anew how to give and receive collaboratively with our brothers and sisters, united in a work that transcends and outlasts us all.

Takeaways

- The church is a people "called-out" (*ekklesia*).
- To be a disciple of Jesus Christ is to be *with* other disciples.
- Redemption means being brought into a people, to have standing, to belong.
- Membership in the church implies mission *with* the church.
- The Bible uses two metaphors to describe the church: family and body. We are a part of God's family, in which we have eternal kinship, and we are members of Christ's body, sharing gifts and working together toward his mission.

4

A Moral Appraisal of
Infertility Treatment

Roughly two years after the miscarriage, John and Lizzy found themselves standing over family photos and a half-assembled adoption portfolio. The adoption agency had provided rudimentary guidelines for organizing their book—tell your story simply and directly. It's not a marketing scheme. When she wasn't at work, sleeping, or walking the dog, Lizzy was with the portfolio. She and John both felt confident about their decision to proceed with adoption. It was a confidence born of prayer and experience. And they were excited about the new venture!

A year and a half earlier John and Lizzy were not looking over family photos, but glossy brochures explaining in inaccessibly technical terms some of their reproductive treatment options. Their eyes gravitated toward familiar words like *hormone*, *artificial*, *laboratory*, *freeze*, and *cycle*. Others, like *surrogacy* and acronyms like *IVF* and *IUI*, were meaningless to them. With the specialist's assistance, however, they were able to grasp a few of the treatments and procedures available to them, at least in theory. The cartoonish images on the brochure offered little insight. Debriefing with one another on the drive home was mostly an exercise in confused repetition.

The fact they could ease into this process slowly was reassuring. "We would begin with some simple tests and assessments," suggested the specialist in script-like cadence, "and then once we identify a potential problem, or mitigating factor, we can then devise a precise treatment regimen." He said that when a treatment produces no result, that's a sign to move along to the next one. The idea was to start with the least invasive option, and then movement up the scale of "involvement" would correspond to John and Lizzy's "comfort level."

Naturally a "mitigating factor" to their "comfort level" was the exorbitant *cost* of these specialized treatments. Elevating to a new phase of treatment also meant escalating to a new price. Excellent as John's insurance benefits were, the policy would not cover many of the optional treatments offered by the clinic. The heaviest costs would be out of pocket. IVF alone could reach upward of twenty thousand dollars. And in the end, despite all the consultations, phases, and costs there was no guarantee of a child. They were "good candidates" for more enhanced reproductive treatments, or so they were told, but John and Lizzy were grounded enough to acknowledge the unfavorable probabilities.

They would proceed incrementally.

Tests were run, scans conducted, samples studied. Lizzy was prescribed a newly developed hormone treatment, supplemented with a range of vitamins she was slightly deficient in. John's tests were unrevealing. They had conceived before, after all. Lizzy later underwent some minor outpatient surgery to remove a cyst from her ovary, to no eventual effect. And here they would stop. They had discussed it before ever commencing with treatment, had sought the advice of family and their pastors, and were resolved not to proceed with IVF or surrogacy.

Three months after submitting their portfolio to the agency John and Lizzy were picking up some produce at the farmers market when they received a surprise phone call: an expecting mother had selected them and wanted very much to meet! Lucy, they came to learn, studied literature at a university. Her pregnancy was an accident and, although persuaded by many of her friends to abort, she felt it was her responsibility to have the baby and then place it with adoptive parents. She said she had reviewed what felt like piles of portfolios before reviewing John and Lizzy's. But when she saw their photos and read their story, she knew they were the ones.

Several months later John and Lizzy smiled broadly at one another as they unlocked the front door, pushed it open, and brought little Grace into their home.

Uncertainty

Infertility reminds us we are not always in control. We are all subject to other powers and realities. Dramatic advances in modern medicine have made it possible for many infertile couples to conceive, although no reproductive treatment enjoys a 100 percent success rate. Yet, despite these advances, we also recognize something profoundly uncertain, even risky, about procreation. Just ask one of the many couples using birth control but who discovered a surprise pregnancy a few weeks later! We haven't the foggiest idea whether "this time" will do the trick. No one is promised children. Couples *hope* for children. Those with hope look to God, the sovereign One and giver of all good gifts. It is possible to see even childlessness as such a gift.

Conception is uncertain. Will sex at the right time of month result in pregnancy? Perhaps. The same uncertainty applies to pregnancy itself. Could it be twins? Boy or girl? Brown eyes or blue? His temperament or hers? We hope and pray for delivery of a healthy baby. "Expecting" is the word we use in this context, and it's right that we do. With only a few grainy ultrasound photos and crudely refined speculations, we wait for children to enter our world. Sometimes babies come when they're ready, and sometimes they need a little coaxing. In either case, the joy of a child's arrival is also tinged with some feeling of relief—the baby is *here* now, safe. At least one reason for this feeling is a corresponding belief, however unconscious, that life in the womb is somehow more uncertain than life outside it. Pregnancy is inescapably pregnant with uncertainties.

At the same time we are not wholly ignorant of the biological conditions and processes of pregnancy. We know more now about the hows, whats, whens, and whys of the human body than at any point in human history. The sheer scale of modern medicine's achievements is hard to capture without resort to hyperbole. Suffice to say, today we are not without remedies or therapies or medications or surgeries or treatments for what ails us. Modern health care has proved it can cure many of our diseases, relieve much of our suffering, reconstruct our appearance, and even extend our life expectancy. Ordinarily we think of health care simply as what we need when we're unwell, and for the most part that is precisely what it is to us.

But medicine can also have other applications, obviously, including treatment of infertility. Couples who experience prolonged infertility often seek the assistance of reproductive specialists. These couples have done all that they know to do—monitoring food intake, stress levels, and natural cycles—and nothing has worked. Like anyone else whose competence has reached its limit, couples understandably solicit the advice and help of an expert. It is what I call the "medical turn." What they need only the specialist can provide.

The purpose of this chapter is to survey several common forms of infertility treatment and offer a moral assessment of them. Medicine has come a long way, as I say, but just because a treatment is available doesn't necessarily mean it should be ventured. Assisted reproductive technologies (ARTs) are complex, as are their ethical implications. My aim here is to make the ethics of artificial reproduction as accessible to readers as possible. Before beginning that appraisal, however, a brief word on a delicate subject: miscarriage.

Miscarriage

Miscarriage is the spontaneous loss of pregnancy before the twentieth week of gestation. Experts estimate that approximately 10 to 20 percent of pregnancies end in miscarriage. The vast majority of miscarriages occur in the very early weeks of pregnancy, usually due to some chromosomal problem with the developing fetus. Miscarriages after week fourteen, on the other hand, are more often attributed to some underlying problem in the mother. Then, after week twenty, the "miscarriage" designation switches to "stillbirth." Although practitioners know far more about the potential causes of miscarriage than they did even a few decades ago, the exact reasons some women are more prone to miscarriage than others remains a subject of considerable study.

The wound of miscarriage is both physical and spiritual. When a child is conceived, so are hopes and expectations. The little one in its safe, nourishing enclosure becomes an object of prayerful concern. A mother's body reacts naturally to this newly formed life, sustaining it and providing the vitality it needs for development. This intimacy between mother and child is exquisite. The mother has no choice as to whether her body will nurture this new life inside. Her body simply reacts.

During gestation mothers share a reciprocal relationship with their child. The umbilical cord linking them is something of a two-way portal. Yes, the mother furnishes far, far more for the child than the child does for the mother, obviously, but the reciprocity they share is crucial to the child's pre- and postnatal development. Mothering begins the moment new life is detected. The connection is physical, hormonal, emotional, and spiritual. Child and mother experience one another.[1] They share life. This directness and intimacy—this *bond*—is also what makes miscarriage so painful and debilitating.

Mothers say they "lost" a child by miscarriage because the term captures precisely how they *feel*. Their little child died. No summary of causes lessens the hurt. Nor does explaining why it happened help a mother fully accept why it happened. Theories are of little consolation. Miscarriage is a tragic fact of human life, a cruel and jarring reminder of the fall. We mourn it and look to a time when it will no longer occur. In the meantime Jesus receives these little ones into his eternal love and peace. Lost to us, in a way, but never lost to him.

Losing a child by stillbirth later in pregnancy is perhaps even more agonizing. A corner is turned after the first trimester, and couples allow themselves a little more hopeful optimism. They announce their pregnancy to family and friends. The loss of a child late in pregnancy is devastating, and to further compound the hardship, in some instances, the mother is required to "deliver" her child either surgically or by induced labor. For many mothers, the experience is physically and emotionally traumatizing: her baby claimed some deeply emotional part of her, and that part died with her baby. What follows, rightly and invariably, is a period of mourning. Some couples may elect to hold memorial services for their little one. It is a time of anguish.

As I have said before, "infertility" applies to a spectrum of experiences. Some infertile couples never conceive, while others conceive but remain unable to carry the child to term. The distinction is an important one because of the unique ways each experience may be treated by medical specialists. The couple that cannot conceive will be prescribed a different regimen or program than the couple that can conceive but cannot bring a child to term. Assessing the ethics of assisted reproductive treatments and technologies requires identifying exact purposes and means of treatment.

Artificial Reproductive Technology

In order to devote ample attention to reproductive technologies presenting the greatest moral challenge, I wish to focus here on two relatively common reproductive technologies: *Intrauterine Insemination* (IUI) and *In Vitro Fertilization* (IVF). By the time these technologies are recommended to a couple, all other less-involved options have been attempted, without success. The specifics of procedures like IUI and IVF are not always clearly conveyed to couples, however, and even when they are, couples sometimes do not wish to know the clinical details.

IUI and IVF constitute more advanced forms of treatment in that they are *extra*bodily. That is, these treatments require special handling, storage, and transport of biological material in a laboratory. Before, a couple's treatments were designed narrowly to aid conception through normal sexual intercourse. Assisted reproductive technologies like IUI and IVF, on the other hand, circumvent sexual intercourse entirely.

To form an accurate Christian ethical assessment of IUI and IVF, it is crucial to understand both the technical procedures themselves and the implications those procedures carry. Too often our posture toward medicine is deferential and admiring. Medicine helps people, we say to ourselves, and the ways it goes about helping people are right because its aim is noble. Medicine does indeed have many laudable aims. But when we subject this particular presumption to closer scrutiny, we must also recognize that means do not always justify ends. There are all sorts of bad ways to go about achieving good ends. We shouldn't lie our way to a promotion, shouldn't wipe out a civilian population to win a battle, and shouldn't inject ourselves with black tar heroine because we want pleasure, to cite a few examples.

In ethics this theory is referred to as *utilitarian*. For the utilitarian, an action is right or wrong in proportion to the positive or negative consequences that action produces. Good actions, in other words, are those that maximize pleasure and minimize pain for the most people. It is easy to see why modern medicine would find this theory attractive. Medicine aspires to heal and to improve the lives of patients—a net positive social contribution.

An overwhelmingly positive social contribution does not also mean, however, that all of medicine's methods and aims are right. Whether a medical practice, procedure, or convention is ethical depends upon much more than some overall social utility. The relevant purposes, methods, and assumptions also deserve consideration.

IUI and IVF are known as assisted reproductive technologies, or ARTs. Reproduction is in this instance assisted technically, mediated by a medical specialist. Intrauterine Insemination is the less complex procedure of the two. With IUI a man's sperm is collected and "washed" to separate sperm from other seminal fluid, at which point the sperm is then inserted directly into the woman's uterus during ovulation, increasing the chances of conception. Inserting sperm directly into the uterus raises the likelihood that at least one sperm will fertilize the egg during ovulation.

Although much less complicated than IVF, IUI still requires involvement of a medical technician to facilitate conception, and thus any couple opting for it should consider the deeper theological question of whether the relation between conception and sex is sacred. Is the manner of procreation as God designed open to amendment? With IUI the amendment is light, one may say, and perhaps a matter of individual conscience.[2] But this question of whether, or to what extent, the method of conception matters to God applies equally to IVF.

In Vitro Fertilization (IVF) is a vastly more complex procedure than IUI, and as such carries more complex ethical implications. The process goes something like this: a man donates his sperm and a woman has eggs harvested, her eggs are fertilized by his sperm in a laboratory (*in vitro* is Latin for "in glass"), and the embryos created are frozen in a clinic until the woman reaches an opportune point in her cycle. In most instances multiple embryos are implanted, on the presumption it increases the chances of at least one embryo implanting successfully. Birth of multiples is for this reason a relatively common occurrence.

A few features of this process deserve further reflection. First, the procreative process is externalized. Procreation is not sexual, strictly speaking, but clinical. Biological material is given over to specialists for fusion and deposit. The natural, intimate link between sexual intercourse and procreation being unfruitful, an artificial method is tried. Artificial fertilization should not, however, try for any *more* than would be tried for in natural procreation; that is, trying for *a* child. A couple should not utilize artificial means either for the express purpose of conceiving multiple children or to genetically enhance the child in any way.[3]

Second, a couple must resolve to set a limit upon the number of eggs to be fertilized. The more embryos created in a lab, the more storage is needed, and the less likely a couple is to have all embryos eventually implanted. It is *essential* that couples have only one egg fertilized and implanted at a time, so as to avoid creating an excess number of embryos a couple may not wish to implant.

Third, what a couple expects to happen through IVF on the front end and what actually transpires are not always congruous. That is the nature of our moral experience in general, of course. We act on expectations of a future that, for a variety of reasons both inside and outside our control, never come to fruition. Expectations may be met or disappointed. It is of great moral importance not to infuse expectations with inevitability.

Lastly, IVF is voluntary and expensive. It is not a treatment in the way vaccines or chemotherapy or angioplasties are treatments. It does not seek to *restore* health. IVF is instead a technical procedure that may or may not furnish couples with children of their own progeny. The average cost of IVF is between fifteen to twenty thousand dollars, a price that upticks with additional services.

Let me expound a bit further on a few of these points. In his prescient book, *Begotten or Made?*, British theologian Oliver O'Donovan cautions against use of IVF for theological reasons. First, there is the matter of IVF's backstory. Clinical IVF became possible because of extensive research trials to test hypotheses and to refine techniques. This research was conducted over the course of many years, and in practice required destruction of untold numbers of human embryos. This was the price to be paid for clinical application. Any Christian couple contemplating IVF must reckon with this backstory.

Second, O'Donovan identifies two "risks" associated with IVF. Natural procreation always involves acceptance of some risk. When a husband and wife conceive, they hope their child will be born healthy and whole. We just don't know for certain what sort of child is coming, or in what condition it will arrive. Pregnancy achieved through IVF, on the other hand, involves acceptance of *enhanced* risk. It is enhanced because of the various artificial mechanisms it involves: specimen gathering, fertilization, freezing, storage, handling, and implantation, not to mention reliance upon various personnel, instruments, and equipment. Compared to natural procreation there is more that could contribute to some complication or malformation to the child. The probability may not be very high, and indeed may even be negligible. But, according to O'Donovan, it's the mere willingness to accept this risk that proves morally decisive. "There is a world of difference," claims O'Donovan, "between accepting the risk of a disabled child (where that risk is imposed upon us by nature) and ourselves *imposing* that risk in pursuit of our own purposes."[4]

Suppose a couple conceives through IVF, and the child is born with an acute cognitive impairment. Are we able to fix responsibility for the impairment with any definiteness? It would seem not, and the inability to do so presents a problem. In what other sphere of our experience, posits O'Donovan, do we observe someone imposing injury on another (in this case on a child) without the prospect of attributing responsibility? Here it cannot be determined when, who, or what may have caused the child's impairment directly, yet a condition of IVF is to accept that such a cause is possible, and ethically speaking, that's all that matters on final account. This is why the mere willingness to accept an enhanced risk itself constitutes moral error.[5]

On the other matter of a potential tension between a couple's early expectations about what IVF may make possible and the real eventualities of their experience, a delicate word is needed. Many Christian couples pursue IVF for reasons they believe consistent with their faith. I know many personally, and I've heard their stories. God has said it is good to have children, they want children, and IVF seems to offer the medical means for realizing their dreams. I have no doubt that a tremendous number of deeply faithful couples opt for IVF with pure intentions.

The moral tension has comparatively little to do with the purity or sincerity of human motivation, however. Of greater concern is the mismatch, common to human experience, between expectations obtaining *prior* to an action and the consequences *brought about* by that action. We use a peculiar word to compliment someone on their flattering appearance, and to our surprise they seem more dejected than cheered up. We pay a hefty fee to enroll in a community course, only to find that we do not have the time for such a commitment after all. We place a family member in assisted living thinking it the best arrangement for him, only to observe his steady slip into depression mere weeks after moving in. Still other examples illustrating the frequent incongruity between expectation and consequence are in great supply. You likely have your own.

As it relates to IVF, the mismatch between expectation and consequence is especially precarious. Suppose a Christian couple opts for IVF after several years of infertility. They are decently informed about the process and ask the clinic to limit fertilization to five eggs. A child is conceived on first implantation, and nine months later a son is born. After a year or so with their little boy, the couple is ready for a second child, and another embryo is implanted successfully. A daughter is born nine months later. All has gone according to plan! So it seemed, until a short ten months after the birth of their daughter, the couple discovers they have conceived *naturally*. (They never figured they'd need contraception!) This turns out not to be an anomaly, because a year after the birth of their third child, they conceive naturally yet again. So, approximately five years after opting for IVF, the couple has two children conceived artificially and two naturally, leaving three embryos still frozen in storage.

The confidence this couple had at the outset to implant all five embryos, once assailed by the pressures of parenting four young children, understandably weakens. Originally they intended to have all five embryos implanted, except now the prospect of having the three remaining embryos implanted strikes them as physically, emotionally, and financially overwhelming. Of course they did not anticipate conceiving children naturally. Of course they did not sufficiently appreciate the range and force of demands children place on parents. Nevertheless, here they are: four children, three frozen embryos, and decisions to make.

Let me be very clear at this point: I do not mean to insinuate that couples who find themselves in the sort of hypothetical position I describe bear permanent and impregnable guilt for their decision. As I said, the initial reasons prompting a couple to opt for IVF are typically formulated on the basis of knowledge available at the time. Had they been fully apprised of the full moral complexity of their decision, perhaps they would not have proceeded in the first place. Even so, they are not relieved of the hard decision of what to do *now* with their frozen embryos. It is of great moral importance to recognize that the future often contains much more contingency than we are often able to appreciate. Some of our projects are realized, and some miscarry; that's an unavoidable feature of human life. Who knows what might happen? That's why the Bible says the proper Christian response to the future is *hope*.

For the Christian couple with frozen embryo(s) they're uncertain about implanting, two options are available: have the embryos implanted as originally intended, or place the embryo(s) up for adoption. Unless the couple faces some extenuating crisis, what Dietrich Bonhoeffer refers to as a "borderline case," frozen embryos should all at some point be implanted in the mother.[6] The extenuating crisis must therefore be very severe indeed; as in, the mother has received a hysterectomy, or, more gravely, has passed away, at which point the biological father may justifiably place embryos for adoption. Such borderline cases aside, couples bear the responsibility to have frozen embryos implanted. A couple's decision in this instance is not whether to have more children; rather, it is acknowledging that they already have children in temporary stasis deserving a chance at full life.

The Christian couple contemplating adopting an embryo is in a slightly different position. Although it is estimated that between five hundred thousand and eight hundred thousand embryos are in frozen storage across the United States, most of which are slated for implantation with biological parents, there are no exact statistics accounting for embryo adoptions nationally. For a variety of reasons, some of these embryos are not finally implanted, and so are either stored as long as a couple leases storage, or they are destroyed or placed for adoption. Because the likelihood of an embryo being destroyed is so disproportionately high, given the surplus number in storage, it is justifiable for a couple to adopt an embryo. The couple adds a child to their family and likewise prevents its destruction.

In allowing for this sort of adoption I wish also to alert couples to two moral problems that may arise. First, the legal language associated with embryo adoption is in many states *transactional*, meaning the contract a donating couple enters with an adopting couple uses terms of *property* exchange. It is imperative that the legal terminology, which in this case is also metaphysically derived, does not in any way suggest an exchange of property. Absence of precise federal statutes on embryo adoptions means that contracts vary from state to state, and to complicate matters further, the legal status of an embryo is a significant issue of debate. Couples considering embryo adoption should do their due diligence both to familiarize themselves with the law and to select a reliable agency.

This leads me to the second cautionary point: the majority of embryo adoption agencies are *for-profit*. Embryos should never be considered a sort of commodity, and any attempt to do so is morally odious. The profit variable in embryo adoptions raises a few other moral concerns that, although not especially prominent today, may become increasingly prominent in the near future, such as the possibility of incentivizing future embryo trading, of individuals partnering with others individuals to produce genetically superior embryo adoption markets, or agencies themselves couching their services in terms of boutique embryo selection. Again, these arrangements do not yet appear to exist, but the ways embryo adoption agencies have constituted and positioned themselves in the market make it a real possibility.

Surrogacy

Technologies associated with IVF also make surrogacy possible. In its standard form "surrogacy" refers to the practice of a couple contracting with a woman to carry their biological child to term and surrender it back to them at birth. This is the most common but by no means the only form a surrogacy contract can take. In fact, it is possible to involve as many as six parties: biological mother, biological father, adopting mother, adopting father, carrying mother, and child that will be born, to say nothing of the IVF clinicians or personnel contributing to recruitment of surrogates and their pre- and postnatal care. Dystopian as the practice may seem, it is now fully mainstream, both within the church and without.

I cannot speak here to all the technicalities of surrogacy or to all the moral repercussions following from it, but do wish to state rather straightforwardly that the dominant transactional form of surrogacy, where a couple remunerates a woman for carrying their child to term, is morally odious. It is indistinguishable from womb rental. Compounding the problem, surrogacy contracts disproportionately favor the contract parents and include few protections for carrying mothers. Even when carrying mothers enter willingly into contract, they remain vulnerable to exploitation. Almost all, for example, include at-will provisions for contracting parents, and for which the carrying mother has no legal recourse.

Alternatively, within the church, the most common form of surrogacy is not transactional but voluntary. A sister offers to carry a child for her sister and brother-in-law, for example, or a close friend for another friend. The carrying mother is compensated only for the expenses accrued by having the child. She is not paid. Why this occurs is understandable, too. Someone wishes to help out a loved one, and such sacrificial generosity seems on first glance beyond reproach.

Nevertheless, as with embryo adoption, the mistake here is in assuming that a pure or altruistic intention is enough to make the action morally right. The exclusive marital bond is, however unwittingly, decoupled for temporary incorporation of another. This is not procreation in the truest sense of the word, but reproduction. Surrogacy proceeds on a parallel assumption that the marital covenant is spiritual but not also material, that it does not make a claim on the human body.[7]

Many surrogates do not anticipate developing an affectionate bond with a child during its gestation and yet do in fact come to form visceral bonds with the child. So here we have a "mother" who brings a child without her own genetic material into the world feeling tangibly bound to it, even to the point of loving and adoring it. Why? Because in utero the "new one" and the mother experience one another in powerful ways.[8] Forming such a natural bond is how God designed it. Surrogates often do not anticipate coming to love the life they're helping bring into the world, and so it comes as no surprise that some of these young women put up a tremendous legal fight to retain custody of children they contracted to give up. Can a surrogate "care" for her developing baby with only her head and without her heart, to simply do her contractual duty, dispassionate to the new one drawing upon her very life and breath? The answer clearly is no, and indeed she shouldn't have to.[9]

Who is the mother of the child born through surrogacy, the surrogate or the woman whose egg was fertilized? The carrying mother or the genetic mother? Our answer will depend upon what we think "mothering" means, of course, but its traditional use strongly suggests that the surrogate has mothered the child to the point of birth. Irrespective of the contract she has formed with another party, the surrogate's body reacts to the child she carries as though it were hers. Her body reacts as designed, as does her child's. In this context the contract is an abstraction. This and similar complexities strongly undercut the Christian ethical legitimacy of surrogacy, no matter how well-meaning someone might be.

Conclusion

The aim of this chapter has been to survey some assisted reproductive technologies, to assess their moral implications, and to offer some moral counsel regarding surrogacy and embryo adoption. We focused primarily on IVF and on the practices and procedures IVF makes possible. I have cautioned against IVF for both theological and moral reasons. If you are contemplating IVF, I pray you take seriously the risks and hazards involved and elect to forgo it, with one proviso. IVF would be acceptable if only one egg were fertilized at a time, never creating more embryos than would be implanted. If you have already proceeded with IVF and as a result face a vexing moral dilemma, I advise not to place embryos up for adoption but instead to have them implanted, then, if necessary, place the child for adoption. That may be terribly hard counsel to accept, I realize; and I do not pretend to understand the struggle you have endured to this point. I can only implore you to seek God's guidance and courage, and to hear again what God has said about his purpose for human beings and their relationships.

I want also to exhort infertile couples not to allow the desire for a biological child to supersede all other biblical, theological, or ethical considerations. I caution against making use of the options above because they presume a certainty about how life will go, when in fact conception and pregnancy are notoriously unpredictable phenomena. Opting for any of the above commits you to risks and dilemmas you would do well to avoid.

Should you choose in favor of them anyway, it will be on the assumption that having a biological child is an end no means could upset, and needless to say, that is not the logic of discipleship but of utility. Speak with others you trust—family, friends, pastors—and do the hard work of listening and thinking and praying. Wise is the one who heeds a sound word of instruction. In Christ are the riches of wisdom, and if anyone lacks wisdom, "let him ask God, who gives generously to all without reproach, and it will be given him" (James 1:5).

Now a brief word for readers who have experienced the pain of infertility: *God loves you, he has not forsaken you, he comes to the afflicted.* Yours is perhaps a unique experience, and although you may often feel alone or despondent, the reassuring truth is that Jesus is familiar with your suffering. "He is actually not far from each one of us," Paul writes (Acts 17:27). In Christ alone is the peace and wisdom to consider present sufferings as not worth comparing to the glory that is to be revealed in us (Rom 8:18).

Takeaways

- Infertility reminds us we are not in control. Conception is uncertain. Nor do we have knowledge of exactly the sort of child that will be born if we do conceive.
- Miscarriage and stillbirth are tragic facts of human existence. They are wounding. These children who pass too early are received into the loving arms of Jesus.
- Of the two artificial reproductive technologies discussed, IUI is the least involved and carries few moral implications.
- IVF carries with it several significant moral implications, including the creation of excess embryos, assumed risks to the child, and expense of treatment.
- IVF may still be morally permissible if couples accept the following in conscience:
  - The remote possibility of impairment or injury to the child.
  - Circumventing natural procreation by artificial means is consistent with God's purpose for sexual union in marriage.

- Only one egg is fertilized and implanted at a time. No excess number of embryos are created or stored.
- Cost of treatment is not overburdening.
- Adoption has been given due consideration, and is not ruled out on the sole basis of wanting a biological child.

- Couples should not place embryos for adoption, unless countervailing circumstances are such that it is the only justifiable course of action.
- Surrogacy is not morally permissible, both for natural and theological reasons.

Appendix

Interview with Patrick and Jennifer Arbo

How long had you been married before trying to have children?
We married in August of 2007 and began trying to conceive in the summer of 2011. Like so many other young couples we know, our timeline was altered by external factors or life circumstances. We believed it was prudent, both spiritually and pragmatically, to wait until graduate school was at least partially completed before starting a family. There would be times when we would revisit that decision, wondering whether we'd actually perceived the Spirit's leading clearly, or perhaps presupposed God's favor. At the time, our hearts didn't entertain the slightest hint of "when I'm good and ready" presumptuousness. But hindsight isn't nearly so kind. It's strange the way that frustrations and anxiety connected to infertility and miscarriage can alter memories or cloud recollections.

When did you first begin to wonder whether you might be experiencing infertility?

After our third miscarriage, what had mostly been an unnamed worry began to take shape and crystalize into fear.

Can you talk about your experience the first time you conceived and parallel it with the feelings you had after the baby miscarried?

They are the perfect antithesis of one another. As a couple, your hearts go from overflowing to desolate, elated to despondent, fleshly to inanimate, and vibrant to monochromatic. This dichotomy was much more pronounced and visceral to us, especially for Jennifer, because, due to the late stage of the pregnancy, the baby had to be delivered naturally, with all the attending risks, complications, and recovery. What was supposed to be this wonderful, life-bringing, and joyful unfolding of events became inversely terrible, spirit-crushing, and empty.

Looking back, what do you wish someone would have said but didn't after the miscarriage? Any word or gesture that meant a lot to you stand out? What do you wish some folks, however well-meaning, had not said?

It is safe to say that, without our families and our brothers and sisters in Christ, the days following Gary's loss would have been almost unbearable. Mercifully, we weren't exposed to many cliché sympathies, though there were some. Regardless of how pure and well-meaning the intentions, the "God wanted another angel up in heaven" suggestion is really a tremendous disservice. Decontextualized Scripture comprised many misguided attempts at comfort as well. Citing God's prophetic promise to the nation of Israel in Jeremiah 29:11 misses the mark at best and is confusing or guilt-inducing at worst. If people are thinking about employing Scripture as a grief-mitigation tool, I would encourage them to assess their ultimate aim. You'll want to avoid—at all costs—any passage in which the chief message you're pressing is: "Well, cheer up," or "It will all be ok in a little while."

Scripture, when it is rightly applied, offers comfort like little else. For example, when two weeks had passed since the delivery of our stillborn son, my mother and father shared 2 Samuel 12:15–23 with me (Patrick) as a subtle encouragement to return to worship and fellowship. I identified with David's grief, his raw brokenness. Likewise, his kingly nobility and resolute leadership called me up and out of grief, to set my face against the prospect of being seen at worship in such a vulnerable, weak state. The following portions of that text became somewhat of a mantra to me: "And he went into the house of the LORD and worshiped . . . 'Can I bring him back again? I shall go to him, but he will not return to me'" (2 Sam. 12:20, 23).

Nor can we overstate the comfort of a friend or family member's "thereness." One of the difficult things for me, and unexpectedly so, was answering the phone. It sounds so simple and ridiculous now, but the enormity of that task in the weeks after the miscarriage was staggering. Voicemails piled up unanswered, though not altogether neglected. I can't express how comforting it was to receive the following sort of message from my brother or best friend, Keith: "Hey buddy. You didn't answer. That's ok, really. I'm going to keep calling because I want you to know that I'm here and that I love you. But, there is *no* pressure to answer the phone. When the time is right for you, ring me or answer, but not a moment sooner. I'll keep leaving you a message every few days, because I just want you to know you're on my heart and in my mind and prayers. I love you, pal." It took me three weeks to slide my thumb across the screen to receive Keith's call; but when I did, it was as though barely a day had passed.

Who was Gary, and how did he change your lives?
Gary was the first child we lost to miscarriage. It didn't take us very long to conceive, which left us with the false assurance that everything was going according to plan. We were overjoyed. We started doing the silly-with-joy things that couples do when expecting. We had a song for Gary, a peculiar language we used to speak to him in the womb, all sorts of plans for the future, and the knowing glances of contentment and peace at the promise of his arrival. Before we knew it (in hindsight, we never felt like we had enough time), we were headed to the OBGYN for the gender reveal. We were nervous, but only about which gender we'd discover. As the final steps in prepping the ultrasound machine were completed, we held hands and our collective breath. We didn't exhale until the next day. As the screen came alive, we could see Gary clearly, but something was off. It is hard to say what it was. I (Patrick) remember that we didn't look at one another for quite some time, unable to admit, even by eye contact, that something was wrong.

The ultrasound technician, bless her, artfully muted the ultrasound audio. No heartbeat was present. She did not want to intimate that anything was amiss until an OBGYN could come in and attempt some different strategies. She said, "I need to go and find your doctor. I need him to double-check some things." Our doctor, a believer and—throughout this situation—the picture of professionalism, entered and somehow sensed that we needed him to acknowledge the thick fear and anxiety in the room. He said, "I want you to know, they asked me to come in and take a look and a listen because they aren't finding a heartbeat. We're going to make absolutely certain, but I want you to know what's going on. Hang in there for me ok, I'll be with you through all of this." He searched, in vain, for what seemed like an eternity. Finally, he withdrew the wand and sighed deeply. "Jennifer, Patrick, I'm sorry but I am unable to find your baby's heartbeat and there are no signs of life." He delivered that news with a tenderness that only comes from experience, compassion, and genuine empathy. He walked us step-by-step through what needed to happen, with haste, but it was all a blur. Only hours later we were at the hospital preparing for inducement. Our stillborn son was born the next morning. We were able to hold him, weep over him, and let him go.

We simply weren't the same people after Gary. It would be easier to explain the ways in which he didn't change our lives than to attempt to explain how he did.

After several more years of infertility, how would you describe your thoughts and feelings? Had you become more calloused or hopeless? Perhaps more mature? Describe your spiritual development during this season.

There were seasons in which we were probably calloused, our hearts chapped with grief from another miscarriage or failed attempt to identify the exact cause of our reproductive issues. There were, however, very sweet seasons in which the soil of our spiritual lives was all the richer for the tilling. Ultimately, we grew closer to God and in intimacy with Jesus. Our spirits deepened as we came to know Christ in his sufferings and treasure his Word all the more fully. Scripture became for us a fixed point of stability when all else was shifting chaos.

Did you have a good church family during this time? Do you feel you were pastored, encouraged, and prayed for? Did you belong to a church small group? Any memories here of a word rightly or wrongly given?

The church was absolutely essential to us. Our miscarriages occurred at intervals that saw us either attending or serving different congregations. We can't say enough about the pastoral care we received. Though we weren't, at the time of any of our miscarriages, involved in a small group (the churches we attended or served were traditional Sunday school and generational ministry-based), we were well-supported by our brothers and sisters in Christ. Some developed an online meal schedule, so that it was easy for those who wanted to bring us a meal to sign up and supply that need. We were incredibly grateful for that. We were visited, prayed for, prayed over, hugged, cried upon, and allowed to cry. Rather than a word rightly or wrongly given, what stands out—thinking back—were those who understood that words were not necessarily beneficial or even required. We remember well, and fondly, those who came simply to sit with us in our grief: to weep, to wipe away tears, to hold.

When did you first begin to contemplate adoption?

We received a call to adopt on a very specific date before we even started trying to conceive. Patrick was attending seminary at Southeastern Baptist Theological Seminary, where he went to chapel twice a week. On this particular day, I (Jennifer) had the day off for Veteran's Day. I was teaching in a local public school and was unable to attend any other chapel service due to my work schedule. On November 11, 2010, Dr. Tony Merida delivered a message on the parallels between the earthly love-act of adoption and foster care, and our adoption as children of God. Patrick and I left that chapel service and immediately began discussing how we felt the Holy Spirit at work in our hearts, calling us to adopt. I don't think either one of us had any idea what that would look like, but God made it clear long before we began having infertility issues. This call was only ever reinforced and strengthened through Scripture.

How did the process unfold?
The summer after receiving what we believed was the call to adopt, we moved back to Tennessee. Patrick had completed a year of seminary on campus, and we moved to be close to family because we were ready to start a family. Patrick was going to keep working on his seminary degree online. He went back to teaching high school, and I continued to teach elementary school. While we knew we wanted to adopt, we both presumed we would have one or two biological children first and then adopt. However, that's not the plan God had in mind. We started the adoption process, on and off, about a year after losing our son. Eventually we were informed about a local organization and decided to try it first. We were matched with a six-year-old boy whom we got to spend time with for about six months. That adoption fell through suddenly, and nothing else worked out with that particular organization. Meanwhile, Patrick accepted the call to vocational ministry, and we moved to South Carolina.

After settling into our new home, we were ready to move forward again with adoption. We began again the *long* paperwork process. I would say that we were a little stubborn when it came to actually committing to the process in its entirety. Although we knew that we were following God's call, it was still somewhat scary. After finally coming to the conclusion that we were all-in, the process gets a little blurred. Unlike many families, we did not have to wait long once all our paperwork was complete. When we filled everything out for the organization, we were very transparent. We were open to a child up to two or three years old, and indicated no other limiting criteria. Once we were approved and placed on "the list," emails began to come in. We received a few emails with opportunities, but none stood out like the email we received detailing very little information on the three blessings who are now our children.

Once it became clear that you were a good match for this sibling group, was there any lingering question of whether to proceed? What memories do you have of that intense period?

We both knew in our hearts that these three precious children were already ours, and the few lingering questions we needed answers for prior to meeting the kids didn't dissuade us from proceeding. We remained guarded until everything was official, of course. There were lots of prayers, seeking guidance of those educated in the field of adoption, and many sleepless nights as we got closer and closer to finalization.

If you had thirty seconds to offer a word of advice to couples considering adoption, what would it be?

Do it! There are so many excuses for not adopting. Having the correct motives is important, but once that has been established, God will pave the way. It may not, and probably won't, be easy. But just wait and see how he will lead and guide you. Finances are one of the major reasons people neglect to move forward. Grants are available to help offset the costs, as well as books providing ideas for fundraisers.

Were you still trying to have biological children? How had your thinking changed about this after adopting the kids, if at all?

We had not thought about trying to have biological children at this point. We were busy learning what it was like to be parents to twin five-year-olds and a two-year-old. As the year began to come to a close, we decided to stop preventing and just leave everything in God's hands. If it was meant to be, we told ourselves, then it would have to be a miracle. We were not trying, but we were not preventing.

What counsel did others give as you were pursuing adoption? Anything you needed to hear—or didn't need to hear?

One narrative in particular can be unproductive, if not altogether destructive. People say: "You know what happens when couples adopt, don't you?" They proceed to inform you conspiratorially about the *fact* of your impending conception. "Everyone," they say flippantly, "who's had trouble conceiving or with miscarriage ends up having a baby after they adopt!" They say this, often completely unaware and oblivious to the pressure, despondency, and improper motivations for adoption this narrative can produce. Pressure ensues because the next pregnancy, if there even is one, bears a weight of expectancy it cannot sustain. Despondency sets in if God grants pregnancy, a miscarriage, stillbirth, or SIDS. Such events leave the couple feeling as if all hope is lost. Jennifer and I were heartbroken to meet a couple—they attended the first information meeting with the Christian adoption agency we worked with—who shamelessly conceded that they were considering adoption as a means only to acquire the post-adoptive "silver bullet." Incidentally, this sort of comment leaves prospective adopting couples feeling shallow and not a little opportunistic. Are we, couples ask themselves incredulously, only doing this to somehow better our chances of conceiving or maintaining a pregnancy to full term? They ask themselves this even though it was in no way part of their adoptive call as received. Pregnancy is not an incantation!

The other comment to avoid is oversimplified assurance that a child-family match will happen "in no time." Many couples wait for several years before being matched with a child or sibling group. Making a comment like this may cause the individual making it to feel better, but will only cause waiting families emotional distress.

In 2016 you learned you were pregnant. How was this similar and/ or dissimilar from your previous experiences? What did you feel?
I will admit that my first thought was not one of elation or excitement, but rather "here we go again," mixed with elation and excitement. We were guarding our hearts.

Describe how your thoughts and feelings changed over the course of the pregnancy.
Jennifer's OB had discovered a protein shortage during routine testing he'd ordered while Jennifer was pregnant with the baby we last miscarried. The test had been done previously, but not *while* Jennifer was pregnant. Jennifer describes her state-of-mind as "cautiously optimistic." I (Patrick) was perhaps more foolhardy.

Would you mind explaining how you felt at Ellie's birth?
A small army of people was praying for us. The entire process could not have gone more smoothly. The inducement produced perfectly pitched contractions. The epidural was, according

to the anesthesiologist, "textbook." The birth was completely without incident. There was a *calm* present to and within us that could only be attributed to the Holy Spirit's active ministry. We don't mind explaining what we felt when we first saw and held Elliott Karis Arbo, but that doesn't mean we're able. There are simply no words to describe the indescribable.

What would you say to the couple who, like you, has gone many years without conceiving a child, but who, unlike you, has still not conceived?
We love you. "The LORD bless you and keep you; the LORD make his face to shine upon you and be gracious to you; the LORD lift up his countenance upon you and give you peace" (Num. 6:24–26).

Notes

Chapter 1: Stories of Infertility and God's Abiding Promise

1. Oliver O'Donovan, *Entering into Rest* (Grand Rapids, MI: Eerdmans, 2017), 145.
2. Dietrich Bonhoeffer, *Discipleship* (Minneapolis: Fortress, 2003), 87n11.

Chapter 2: Christian Discipleship and Human Affection

1. For more on this line of thinking about discipleship see Dietrich Bonhoeffer's *Discipleship* (Minneapolis: Fortress Press, 2003).
2. Bonhoeffer, *Discipleship* (Minneapolis: Fortress, 2003, 87n11.
3. Karen Swallow Prior, "Called to Childlessness: The Surprising Ways of God," ERLC, March 6, 2017, https://erlc.com/resource-library/articles /called-to-childlessness-the-surprising-ways-of-god/.

Chapter 3: The Vitality and Consolation of the Church

1. For more on the meaning and beauty of God's covenant see Peter Gentry and Stephen Wellum's *Kingdom through Covenant: A Biblical-Theological Understanding of the Covenants* (Wheaton, IL: Crossway: 2012).
2. Oliver O'Donovan, *Desire of the Nations* (Cambridge: Cambridge University Press: 1999), 36.
3. Jonathan Franzen, *The Corrections* (New York: Picador: 2002), 267.
4. See Augustine's *City of God*, trans. R. Dyson (Cambridge: Cambridge University Press, 1998) and Oliver O'Donovan, *Common Objects of Love* (Grand Rapids, MI: Eerdmans, 2009).

Chapter 4: A Moral Appraisal of Infertility Treatment

1. I have benefited tremendously from James Mumford's work on the bond of mother and child. See especially *Ethics at the Beginning of Life* (Oxford: Oxford University Press, 2015).

2. It should go without saying, however, that use of sperm other than the husband's is tantamount to adultery and thus a violation of the marital bond.

3. As this book came to completion, news broke of the first successful gene editing of human embryos. This achievement, if reproducible, takes medical research one step closer to procedural genetic modification of embryos. Such modifications could theoretically apply to treatment of inheritable diseases, like Huntington's disease, sickle cell anemia, or Down syndrome. How to determine precisely which diseases should be edited out of the species as a matter of course is not yet a subject of focused ethical discussion—nor is the more disconcerting possibility created by this new technology: *enhancement*. It may soon be possible for parents to design their child by selecting from a boutique of traits. For more about the first successful editing of a human embryo, see Steve Connor, "First Human Embryos Edited in U.S.," *MIT Technology Review*, July 26, 2018, https://www.technologyreview.com/s/608350/first-human-embryos-edited-in-us/.

4. Oliver O'Donovan, *Begotten or Made?* (Oxford, UK: Clarendon Press, 1984), 83.

5. O'Donovan goes on to show that in the process of IVF, begetting is replaced by artificial making. This is of significant moral consequence. As another Christian thinker, Robert Spaemann, has remarked: "Our beginning is not the work of human hands, but rather occurs by way of a human act that does not take the creating of a product as its primary goal. Only in this way can a human being come to life in her own right, 'by nature,' as creature of God, or at least of nature, yet not of her parents. Genitum non factum, begotten not thrown together in a test-tube, and therefore without the right to demand justification for her existence." See "Human Dignity," in *Essays in Anthropology*, trans. G. DeGraf and J. Mumford (Eugene, OR: Wipf and Stock, 2010), 68.

6. Dietrich Bonhoeffer, *Ethics* (Minneapolis: Fortress Press, 2008).

7. This discounting or disregarding of materiality is actually a deeply gnostic tendency. Though the early church powerfully confronted Gnosticism, this heresy reincarnates itself at peculiar times in church history. To illustrate, gnostics rejected Christ's humanity, that God

took on flesh, because they believed that the simple fact of materiality would profane God.

8. See Mumford's *Ethics at the Beginning of Life.*

9. See my article "Surrogacy and the Making of Modern Families," ELRC, June 15, 2015, https://erlc.com/resource-library/articles/surrogacy-and -the-making-of-modern-families/.

General Index

Scripture Index

Scripture Index